2009
YEAR BOOK OF
**PLASTIC AND
AESTHETIC SURGERY**™

# The 2009 Year Book Series

Year Book of Anesthesiology and Pain Management™: Drs Chestnut, Abram, Black, Gravlee, Lee, Mathru, and Roizen

Year Book of Cardiology®: Drs Gersh, Cheitlin, Elliott, Graham, Sundt, and Waldo

Year Book of Critical Care Medicine®: Drs Dellinger, Parrillo, Balk, Bekes, Dorman, and Dries

Year Book of Dentistry®: Drs Olin, Belvedere, Davis, Henderson, Johnson, Ohrbach, Scott, Spencer, and Zakariasen

Year Book of Dermatology and Dermatologic Surgery™: Drs Thiers and Lang

Year Book of Diagnostic Radiology®: Drs Osborn, Abbara, Birdwell, Elster, Gardiner, Levy, Manaster, Oestrich, and Rosado de Christenson

Year Book of Emergency Medicine®: Drs Hamilton, Handly, Quintana, Werner, and Bruno

Year Book of Endocrinology®: Drs Mazzaferri, Bessesen, Clarke, Howard, Kennedy, Leahy, Meikle, Molitch, Rogol, and Schteingart

Year Book of Gastroenterology™: Drs Lichtenstein, Dempsey, Drebin, Jaffe, Katzka, Kochman, Makar, Morris, Osterman, Rombeau, and Shah

Year Book of Hand and Upper Limb Surgery®: Drs Chang and Steinmann

Year Book of Medicine®: Drs Barkin, Berney, Frishman, Garrick, Loehrer, Phillips, and Khardori

Year Book of Neonatal and Perinatal Medicine®: Drs Fanaroff, Ehrenkranz, and Stevenson

Year Book of Neurology and Neurosurgery®: Drs Kim and Verma

Year Book of Obstetrics, Gynecology, and Women's Health®: Drs Dungan and Shulman

Year Book of Oncology®: Drs Loehrer, Arceci, Glatstein, Gordon, Hanna, Morrow, and Thigpen

Year Book of Ophthalmology®: Drs Rapuano, Cohen, Eagle, Flanders, Hammersmith, Myers, Nelson, Penne, Sergott, Shields, Tipperman, and Vander

Year Book of Orthopedics®: Drs Morrey, Beauchamp, Huddleston, Peterson, Swiontkowski, and Trigg

Year Book of Otolaryngology-Head and Neck Surgery®: Drs Balough, Gapany, Keefe, and Sindwani

Year Book of Pathology and Laboratory Medicine®: Drs Raab, Parwani Bejarano, and Bissell

Year Book of Pediatrics®: Dr Stockman

2009

# The Year Book of PLASTIC AND AESTHETIC SURGERY™

Editor-in-Chief

**Stephen H. Miller, MD, MPH**

*Voluntary Clinical Professor of Surgery and Family Medicine, University of California at San Diego, San Diego, California*

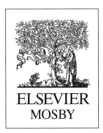

ELSEVIER
MOSBY

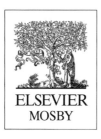

ELSEVIER
MOSBY

*Vice President, Continuity:* John A. Schrefer
*Developmental Editor:* Ruth Malwitz
*Production Manager, Electronic Year Books:* Donna M. Skelton
*Electronic Article Manager:* Travis L. Ross
*Illustrations and Permissions Coordinator:* Linda S. Jones

**2009 EDITION**

Printed in the United States of America
Composition by TnQ Books and Journals Pvt Ltd, India
Printing/binding by Sheridan Books, Inc.

Editorial Office:
Elsevier
1600 John F. Kennedy Blvd.
Suite 1800
Philadelphia, PA 19103-2899

International Standard Serial Number: 1535-1513
International Standard Book Number: 978-1-4160-5736-9

# Editorial Board

# Table of Contents

# Journals Represented

Journals represented in this YEAR BOOK are listed below.

Acta Oto-Laryngologica
Aesthetic Plastic Surgery
Aesthetic Surgery Journal
American Journal of Ophthalmology
Annals of Plastic Surgery
Annals of Surgery
Annals of Thoracic Surgery
Archives of Facial Plastic Surgery
Burns
Dermatology
European Journal of Plastic Surgery
Head & Neck
International Journal of Oral and Maxillofacial Surgery
Journal of American College of Surgeons
Journal of Applied Physiology
Journal of Hand Surgery
Journal of Orthopaedic Trauma
Journal of Pediatric Surgery
Journal of Plastic, Reconstructive & Aesthetic Surgery
Journal of Otolaryngology
Journal of Surgical Research
Microsurgery
Ophthalmology
Otolaryngology-Head and Neck Surgery
Plastic and Reconstructive Surgery
Surgery

To facilitate the use of the YEAR BOOK OF PLASTIC AND AESTHETIC SURGERY as a reference tool, all illustrations and tables included in this publication are now identified as they appear in the original article. This change is meant to help the reader recognize that any illustration or table appearing in the YEAR BOOK OF PLASTIC AND AESTHETIC SURGERY may be only one of many in the original article. For this reason, figure and table numbers will often appear to be out of sequence within the YEAR BOOK OF PLASTIC AND AESTHETIC SURGERY.

# Introduction

This past year has been one of momentous change for the YEAR BOOK of PLASTIC AND AESTHETIC SURGERY and its associate editors. We have plunged, or should I say "plugged" into the electronic age with the able assistance and guidance of the YEAR BOOK staff. Although the learning curve during the transition has been steep, the associate editors and the editorial and information technology staff at Elsevier have been supportive and responsive to the needs and suggestions to make the process more user-friendly. The latter have done a fine job in helping to launch this new YEAR BOOK and I congratulate them on their support and efforts to learn and adapt to the new system. As a result, I believe the 2009 YEAR BOOK is now a timelier and more up-to-date reference than it has been in the past. While a major emphasis has been directed toward the electronic version, Elsevier is committed to continue publishing an annual hard copy version as long as there is adequate interest and need for that type of format by you, the readers.

The electronic version of the YEAR BOOK series and by series I mean all 27 subjects, including the YEAR BOOK of PLASTIC AND AESTHETIC SURGERY, called eClips Consult, has been populated with all of the articles selected from the 2006 volumes to present. With the help of an expert panel of plastic surgeons, articles can now be categorized according to evidence-based medical principles and importance to plastic surgeons. Some of the more exciting aspects of the new electronic version include: the opportunity for the associate editors to select and comment on articles as soon as they are published in a journal, the opportunity for readers to provide instant feedback about each article, the ability to perform detailed searches of past YEAR BOOK content, and finally, the option for subscribers to build a profile of those areas within the specialty of plastic surgery which are of personal interest to them.

This year's YEAR BOOK is one of the more eclectic I have helped to edit. Overall, the selections have begun to reflect efforts to report on multi-centered collaborative studies, the international plastic surgery community, the economics of plastic surgery, and the new paradigms of plastic surgery education.

We have had several changes in the associate editorial staff and wish to thank Dr Scott Bartlett for his many years of service. We will miss his fine contributions and cogent critiques of articles in the area of congenital plastic surgery. A replacement will be named shortly.

Dr Peter McKinney has stepped down as the associate editor primarily responsible for aesthetic surgery but will continue to provide his insights for that section as a contributing guest editor. Dr Karol Gutowski of the University of Wisconsin will assume primary responsibility for this section.

Ruth Malwitz, our fine staff editor, will be leaving the YEAR BOOK of PLASTIC AND AESTHETIC SURGERY during this coming year. We wish her well in her new endeavors. Barbara Cohen-Kligerman, a senior editor at Elsevier, will be assuming responsibility for the YEAR BOOK of PLASTIC AND AESTHETIC SURGERY. Ms Cohen-Kligerman is also senior staff editor of the *Clinics in Plastic Surgery.*

**Stephen H. Miller, MD, MPH**

# 1 Congenital

## Auricular Malformations

### A 20-Year Experience with the Brent Technique of Auricular Reconstruction: Pearls and Pitfalls

Osorno G (Natl Univ of Colombia, Bogotá)
*Plast Reconstr Surg* 119:1447-1463, 2007

*Background.*—The surgical treatment of 291 patients with auricular deformities is reported. This series includes correction of acquired defects in 15 patients and congenital malformations in the remaining 276. In the latter group, 222 had unilateral microtia, 38 had bilateral microtia, and 16 deformities were attributable to failed reconstructions.

*Methods.*—Technical details are given on the planning and executing of operations, including the following: positioning of the reconstructed ear; unconventional lobule transposition for selected patients with facial microsomia; costal cartilage harvesting; framework construction with absorbable sutures; tragus and auricular sulcus construction; and secondary reconstructions with temporal fascial flaps, radical framework revision using the same skin pocket, and total reconstructions with costal cartilage grafts using the original skin envelope.

*Results.*—A total of 326 ears were reconstructed in 291 patients using autogenous costal cartilage: 222 in unilaterally affected microtia patients, 73 in 38 bilaterally affected microtia patients, 16 secondary reconstructions of microtia patients, and 15 in acquired deformities. Two hundred sixty-four of the 291 patients (90.7 percent) were examined at least 1 year after completing treatment. In the remaining 27 patients (9.3 percent), follow-up was not possible for several reasons. Surgery-related complications (hematoma, skin loss, and infection) totaled 1.9 percent. Hypertrophic scars and keloids, with important aesthetic consequences, were 5.3 percent.

*Conclusions.*—Consistently good results were associated with progressive experience and favorable conditions (i.e., isolated type II or III microtia, appropriate amount and quality of costal cartilage, and thin and elastic auricular skin). Recognizing unfavorable conditions helped with sound preoperative planning and discussion of expectations with patients and families.

▶ This is a marvelous report, documenting a large personal experience of reconstructions of congenital and acquired ear deformities from a single surgeon, from Bogota, Columbia. The author borrows from Brent's work, but adds some fresh ideas, based on his own personal experiences. It is a much welcome follow-up to a previous paper by the author, published in Plastic and Reconstructive Surgery in 1999.[1] The ingenuity and experience of the author, in being able to deal with unfavorable preoperative conditions, is evident and worthy of careful consideration.

I am particularly intrigued with the author's use of absorbable sutures to construct the ear framework, and although some of the patients have been followed as long as 4 years, I believe a longer follow-up will be necessary.

**S. H. Miller, MD, MPH**

*Reference*

1. Osorno G. Autogenous rib cartilage reconstruction of congential ear defects: report of 110 cases with Brent's technique. *Plast Reconstr Surg.* 1999;104:1951.

---

### Retrospective Analysis of the Farrior Technique for Otoplasty

Scharer SA, Farrior EH, Farrior RT (Jacksonville Otolaryngology & Facial Plastic Surgery, PA, FL; private practice, Tampa, FL)
*Arch Facial Plast Surg* 9:167-173, 2007

---

*Objective.*—To evaluate clinical outcomes and patient satisfaction following otoplasty for surgical correction of protruding or prominent ears using the Farrior technique.

*Methods.*—This was a retrospective study of patients undergoing cosmetic otoplasty with the Farrior method at a private facial plastic surgery practice in Tampa, Fla. The study population comprised 75 subjects, desiring operative correction of auricular deformities, by one of the authors (E.H.F.) over the past 15 years. The subjects (40 male and 35 female) ranged in age from 5 to 68 years, with a mean age of 23.9 years. Clinical follow-up ranged from 1 day to 7 years 2 months, with a mean duration of 1 year 5 days. The Farrior otoplasty is a graduated technique that combines elements of cartilage sculpting, suturing, and conchal setback procedures, and stresses a patient-specific, anatomy-directed approach. This method was first introduced in the literature in 1959 by the senior author (R.T.F.) and is continued to the present day by his son (E.H.F.). Main outcome measures included satisfactory correction of auricular deformity, incidence of postoperative complications, and degree of patient satisfaction with the procedure. These outcomes were compared with that of other otoplasty techniques and long-term studies in the literature.

*Results.*—Of the 75 patients who underwent otoplasty via the Farrior technique over the last 15 years, bilateral otoplasties were performed in 69 (92%). Of the cases, 69 (92%) were primary procedures, with revision otoplasties constituting 6 (8%) of the total. A combination of conchal cartilage reduction, cartilage scoring, and mattress suturing was the most frequently used maneuver (47 cases [63%]). Most cases were performed using local anesthesia (n = 62 [83%]), with 18 (24%) of all cases having adjunctive procedures at the time of the otoplasty. No major complications (large hematoma, tissue necrosis, gross deformity, or significant wound infection) were documented. A total of 40 minor complications were observed in 29 patients, with suture extrusion and persistent auricular protrusion being the most common (occurring in 14 [19%] and 17 [23%] cases, respectively). Overall, 11 patients required revision surgery (9 for protrusion, 1 for hypertrophic scar, and 1 for cartilaginous callus). A majority of positive responses on an anonymous patient survey reflects a high degree of patient satisfaction with the procedure and results.

*Conclusions.*—The Farrior otoplasty is a graduated technique that has met with clinical success over the years. It combines elements of cartilage shaping and suturing procedures, and as such, is susceptible to complications such as suture extrusion and auricular protrusion that are ascribed to similar otoplasty methods described in the literature. It allows for a directed approach to correct the causative anatomic defects, while maintaining a natural appearance. While further research and long-term analyses are encouraged, this technique remains

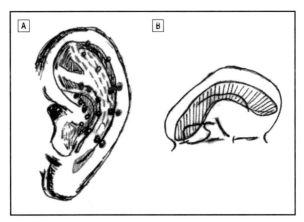

FIGURE 1.—Diagram of maneuvers commonly used in the Farrior otoplasty. A, Placement of mattress sutures and scoring incisions along the posterior surface, seen from the anterior view. Note the elliptical excision of lateral conchal cartilage along the conchal rim and trimming of cauda helicis inferiorly. No incisions through cartilage are made in the region of the superior crus. B, "Elliptical dumbbell" excision of skin seen from the posterior view. (Courtesy of Scharer SA, Farrior EH, Farrior RT. Retrospective analysis of the Farrior technique for otoplasty. *Arch Facial Plast Surg.* 2007; 9:167-173.)

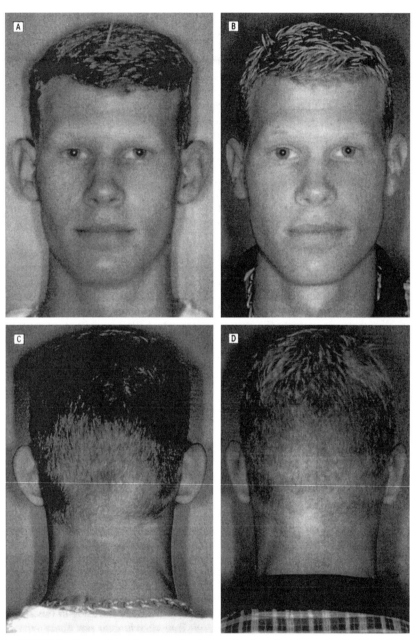

FIGURE 2.—Preoperative and postoperative photographs of a male patient undergoing bilateral otoplasty via the Farrior technique. A, Preoperative frontal view; B, postoperative frontal view; C, preoperative rear view; and D, postoperative rear view. (Courtesy of Scharer SA, Farrior EH, Farrior RT. Retrospective analysis of the Farrior technique for otoplasty. *Arch Facial Plast Surg.* 2007; 9:167-173.)

a valuable component of a facial plastic surgeon's armamentarium (Figs 1 and 2).

▶ This is a composite technique, which combines multiple approaches, and the authors provide us with a 15-year follow-up, although the procedure has been around for nearly 40 years. It reiterates the principles of otoplasty and that there may be multiple deformities requiring a variety of approaches in the same patient. It also provides us with statistics, as to the most frequent complications requiring reoperation.

**P. W. McKinney, MD, CM**

---

**Effects of Different Suture Materials on Cartilage Reshaping**
Cagici CA, Cakmak O, Bal N, et al (Baskent Univ, Faculty of Medicine, Ankara, Turkey)
*Arch Facial Plast Surg* 10:124-129, 2008

---

*Objective.*—To examine the effects of different suture materials and suturation techniques on cartilage reshaping in a rabbit model.

*Methods.*—Twenty-two rabbits were used. Posterior skin flaps were elevated, and 4 cartilage struts were prepared on each auricula. Each strut was bent at its midpoint, and the skin under the bent area was elevated only in 1 side. The strut was sutured either with catgut, polyglactin 910, polydioxanone, or polypropylene sutures. Anteriorly, the suture was passed subcutaneously on 1 side, while transcutaneously on the other. Animals were killed at the first and fourth months. The shape of the struts was macroscopically evaluated. Inflammation and foreign body reaction around the suture were examined under light microscopy.

*Results.*—Maintenance of shape with all suture materials was significantly lower in the transcutaneously sutured group than in the subcutaneously sutured group. Because of high rates of suture loss in the transcutaneously sutured group, further evaluations on cartilage tissue were made only in subcutaneously sutured group. Success rate in maintenance of shape was similarly high in the polydioxanone, polyglactin 910, and polypropylene suture groups; however, it was significantly lower in the catgut suture group.

*Conclusion.*—Long-lasting absorbable suture materials are as effective as nonabsorbable ones, and the subcutaneous technique is more effective than the transcutaneous technique.

▶ I have always thought that permanent sutures are not needed because they cut through the tissue in the long run and lose their effect. Therefore, like a good houseguest, they should do their job and leave. Hence, I have favored the dissolvable sutures. The authors demonstrate that permanent sutures do not lose their effectiveness; this may be from the deposition of collagen so that wires of scar suspend the tissue. The question still remains: Is this collagen deposited before the permanent sutures cut through the tissue or after, therefore being less effective?

P. W. McKinney, MD, CM

# 2  Neoplastic, Inflammatory and Degenerative Conditions

## Benign and Malignant Tumors of the Skin, Head, and Neck

**An approach to managing non-melanoma skin cancer of the nose with mucosal invasion: our experience**
Chiummariello S, Dessy LA, Buccheri EM, et al (Univ La Sapienza, Rome; et al)
*Acta Oto-Laryngol* 128:915-919, 2008

*Conclusions.*—The absence of recurrences after final nasal reconstruction demonstrates the reliability of our three-stage strategy and the necessity to delay nasal reconstruction, focusing attention on oncological safety for nasal non-melanoma skin cancer (NMSC) with mucosal invasion.

*Objectives.*—To validate a therapeutic strategy aimed at oncological safety and minimization of possible recurrences after full-thickness excision of nasal NMSC with mucosal invasion. The strategy was divided into three stages: surgical excision with clinically safe perilesional skin margins and extemporary frozen section histological control; 8–15 months follow-up leaving the nasal defect unreconstructed with a 'wait and see' strategy; new extemporary histological control of defect margins and, if negative, definitive reconstruction.

*Patients and Methods.*—Twenty patients affected by nasal NMSC with mucosal invasion were treated and followed up.

*Results.*—Basal cell carcinoma was the most common lesion (75%), followed by squamous cell carcinoma (25%). Ultrasonography excluded lymphatic involvement for SCC. Before final reconstruction, extemporary histological examination revealed the presence of tumour cells in three patients. After tumour extirpation, these patients were resubmitted to a new follow-up period before reconstruction. No recurrences were

7

observed after definitive nasal reconstruction in all patients during the 5-year follow-up.

▶ This seems like a very long run for a short slide. One wonders whether the same result could have been achieved if the surgeons, in the absence of the availability of Mohs', removed the tumors with a wider margin than described by them and subjected the material to frozen section evaluation using the same clock wise locations as they did for their follow-up biopsies.

**S. H. Miller, MD, MPH**

---

**Microscopic Margins and Results of Surgery for Dermatofibrosarcoma Protuberans**

Popov P, Böhling T, Asko-Seljavaara S, et al (Helsinki Univ Hosp; Univ of Helsinki)
*Plast Reconstr Surg* 119:1779-1784, 2007

---

*Background.*—Dermatofibrosarcoma protuberans is a rare, low-grade sarcoma of the skin with a tendency to recur locally after inadequate excision. Treatment has traditionally been wide excision with a 2- to 3-cm gross margin. Because of the variable results presented in mainly retrospective reports, it has been queried whether local control can be as good with conventional surgery as with micrographic surgery.

*Methods.*—Forty patients with dermatofibrosarcoma protuberans treated by surgical excision, were operated on at our center from 1987 to 2001. Data were recorded prospectively. Twenty-seven patients presented with a primary tumor and 13 with a locally recurrent tumor primarily operated on elsewhere. Gross and histologic margins were studied in detail.

*Results.*—At a mean follow-up of 40 months, there were no recurrences. Thirty-four patients required single, five patients two, and one patient three operations before the margins were adequate (mean, 1.2 stages per patient). Twenty-three patients (58 percent) needed reconstructions. Tumor-free margins were obtained in 39 patients. The average thickness of surgical gross margins was 3.1 cm; histologically defined margins averaged 1.6 cm.

*Conclusions.*—Good local control can be achieved with wide surgery. Histologic tumor-free margins differ greatly from gross margins and are difficult to assess clinically and macroscopically. Careful postoperative histologic examination with margins measured in millimeters should be carried out to define the adequacy of excision in all directions. On average, a 1.6-cm histologic margin was adequate for complete local control. Most patients can be operated on in one stage. Reconstructions are often needed.

▶ Recent articles have suggested that Mohs micrographic surgery is the treatment of choice for Dermatofibrosarcoma protuberans (DFSP). These authors have been able to show that more traditional surgical techniques (ie, wide surgical excision) are as effective as, and perhaps more efficient, than the Mohs approach, provided certain guidelines regarding histologic examination and required reoperation are followed. By "as effective as", I mean that the "cure" rate is the same or better with the traditional approach. By "more efficient", I mean that the traditional method (using the authors principles) requires fewer operations. I have always favored the traditional approach, but now I have objective evidence to back up my choice.

**R. L. Ruberg, MD**

---

**125I seed implant brachytherapy-assisted surgery with preservation of the facial nerve for treatment of malignant parotid gland tumors**
Zhang J, Zhang JG, Song TL, et al (Peking Univ School, Hosp of Stomatology, Beijing, China)
*Int J Oral Maxillofac Surg* 37:515-520, 2008

---

The surgical treatment of malignant parotid gland tumors, combined with 125I seed implant brachytherapy and preservation of the facial nerve is described. Tumor and parotid gland resection with preservation of the facial nerve was carried out in 12 patients with malignant parotid gland tumors. 125I seeds were implanted into the target area intra- or postoperatively. The extent of regional control of the tumor was followed up, and facial nerve function was evaluated. None of the patients had tumor recurrence during the follow-up period of 50–74 months (median follow-up period, 66 months). Facial nerve function had recovered to normal by 6 months postoperatively in all patients. A limited surgical resection combined with 125I seed implant brachytherapy is therefore considered to be an alternative treatment for local control of malignant parotid gland tumors with preservation of the facial nerve.

▶ Excision of malignant, parotid gland tumors involving the facial nerve, are prone to result in sacrifice of the nerve and, not infrequently, local recurrence of the malignancy.[1] Although reconstructive microneurosurgical is often performed at the time of the initial resection, the effect of this on recurrence rates is not well documented, and the return of facial nerve function is often delayed and may be incomplete. Treatment of parotid malignancy, using external beam radiation, may be helpful in those instances in which the tumor is radiosensitive, but with a great deal of morbidity. The authors' proposal to maintain facial nerve function and treat with 125I seeds is appealing. The relatively long-term follow-up certainly would seem to support a larger study and more careful distribution of patients, in accord with documentation of actual involvement of the facial nerve. It is important to document that the tumors actually involve the facial nerve and not just the nerve or its branches in an inflammatory response. Furthermore, it is also important to differentiate the types of tumors, their grades of malignancy, and the timing for the measurement of outcomes. They surely differ for the mixed bag of parotid tumors presented in this series.

**S. H. Miller, MD, MPH**

*Reference*

1. Spiro JD, Spiro RH. Cancer of the parotid gland: role of the 7th nerve preservation. *World J Surg.* 2003;27:863-867.

# Head and Neck Reconstruction

## Comparison of reconstructive procedures in primary versus secondary mandibular reconstruction

Andrade WN, Lipa JE, Novak CB, et al (Univ of Toronto, Ontario; Univ Health Network, Toronto, Ontario; et al)
*Head Neck* 30:341-345, 2008

*Background.*—Few reports have compared reconstructive outcomes of primary versus secondary mandibular reconstruction.

*Methods.*—A retrospective chart review was performed on 149 patients following primary ($n = 110$) and secondary reconstruction ($n = 39$).

*Results.*—There was no statistically significant difference in patient demographics between the 2 groups. The secondary reconstruction mandibular defects were more extensive; significantly more involved the condyle or the central portion of the mandible. The vascularized fibular flap was most commonly used (primary 82%, secondary 69%). The overall complication rate was similar in both groups. There was no statistical difference in the frequency of complications between the primary or secondary reconstruction groups (acute, $p = .40$; late, $p = .17$).

*Conclusions.*—Success in secondary mandibular reconstruction could be achieved utilizing a range of osseous free flaps, and there was no increased rate of complications compared with primary mandibular reconstructions.

▶ This is an interesting, retrospective study, comparing some outcomes after primary versus secondary mandibular reconstruction using free osseous flaps and performed in a single institution. It was surprising to read that, overall, the complication rate in the 2 groups of patients was not significantly different, although, the secondary reconstructions involved more extensive defects, often involving defects of the central segment or condyle, and included patients with osteoradionecrosis and complications secondary to their primary ablative resection. No doubt, these good results are a testament to the skillful, collaborative surgical efforts of the authors. One of the issues, which needs further clarification, is a statement that the length of stay (LOS) in both groups was virtually the same. This fails to take into account that the secondary reconstructive patients have already had a hospital stay for their primary procedure. This information, clearly, is important when one considers the total costs for treatment in these patients must, of course, consider both ablation and reconstruction. It would be beneficial for the authors to continue to add more patients, increase the length of follow up, and expand this study to compare functional and aesthetic outcomes.

**S. H. Miller, MD, MPH**

### Reconstruction of orbital floor and maxilla with divided vascularised calvarial bone flap in one session

Bilen BT, Kılınç H, Arslan A, et al (Inönü Univ, Malatya, Turkey)
*J Plast Reconstr Aesthetic Surg* 59:1305-1311, 2006

We present four cases which underwent reconstruction of orbital floor and anterior maxillary wall, with a vascularised bone flap, following partial maxillectomy. After tumour resections, superficial temporal artery (STA) and vein based calvarial bone flaps from the outer tabula were prepared. Without disrupting the integrity of fascia and periosteum, the bone was separated into two segments in the same direction as the blood flow, and one is 3 cm and the other 5 cm. The two bone segments were transferred as one single flap, and one segment of the flap was used to reconstruct the orbital floor and the other for reconstruction of the anterior maxillary wall. Since two cases had large skin defects, lateral frontal skin, to which the frontal branch of the STA supplies blood, was incorporated into the flaps. Functional and aesthetic results were satisfactory at the end of 8–20 months follow-up. This technique allowed reconstruction of the orbital floor and anterior maxillary wall and, even, skin defects with a single pedicled flap in one session (Figs 3 and 5).

▶ This is a unique modification for the use of a vascularised split calvarial flap to reconstruct bony defects of the orbital floor and anterior maxilla

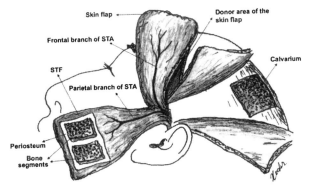

FIGURE 3.—Schematic illustration of divided vascularised calvarial bone flap, including forehead skin island flap based on frontal branch of STA. (Reprinted from Bilen BT, Kılınç H, Arslan A, et al. Reconstruction of orbital floor and maxilla with divided vascularised calvarial bone flap in one session. *J Plast Reconstr Aesthetic Surg.* 2006;59:1305-1311, with permission from The British Association of Plastic Surgeons.)

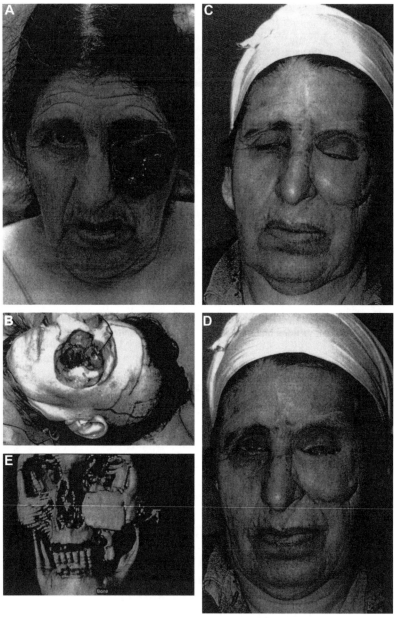

FIGURE 5.—Case 2. A: Pre-operative view of SCC with infraorbital invasion. B: Intra-operative view. Note the defect after partial maxillectomy, including the orbital floor rim, anterior maxillary wall, lower eyelid, infraorbital skin and lateral and medial canthus. C, D: Post-operative view four months after surgery. Note symmetry of inferior orbital rim and anterior maxillary wall without dystopia, enophthalmos and ptosis. Redness of eye is noted. E: Three-dimensional computerized tomography, six months after surgery. Note the orbital and maxillary integrity. (Reprinted from Bilen BT, Kılınç H, Arslan A, et al. Reconstruction of orbital floor and maxilla with divided vascularised calvarial bone flap in one session. *J Plast Reconstr Aesthetic Surg.* 2006;59:1305-1311, with permission from The British Association of Plastic Surgeons.)

(bidirectional bony reconstruction), based on a single pedicle. It was used, successfully, in 4 cases. Basing the flap on the superficial temporal artery system allows one to incorporate lateral frontal skin if necessary to fill associated skin defects. This concept should certainly prove useful for the surgeon responsible for reconstructing these difficult maxillary and periorbital defects.

**S. H. Miller, MD, MPH**

## Medial Sural Artery Perforator Flap For Tongue And Floor Of Mouth Reconstruction

Chen S-L, Chen T-M, Dai N-T, et al (Natl Defense Med Ctr, Taipei, Taiwan)
*Head Neck* 30:351-357, 2008

*Background.*—The radial forearm flap is frequently considered the first choice for tongue reconstruction, but the disadvantages of donor site morbidity are well known. The search for another thin skin flap as an alternative has led to the application of the medial sural artery perforator flap.

*Methods.*—We used 12 medial sural artery perforator flaps to reconstruct tongue and floor of mouth following cancer ablation. We paid attention to the major perforator (vein ≥ 1 mm) as the vascular relay.

*Results.*—Most flaps were raised with a single perforator. The size of the skin paddle varied from 9 cm × 5 cm to 14 cm × 12 cm. The mean thickness of the flap was 5.2 mm. We reexplored 1 patient for venous insufficiency and could not salvage the flap.

*Conclusions.*—The thin medial sural artery perforator flap permits high accuracy of tongue restoration and reduces the morbidity at the donor site.

▶ The medial sural artery flap was originally described in 2001 in *Plastic and Reconstructive Surgery.*[1] Subsequently, it has been used primarily for reconstruction of extremity wounds. These authors report its use as a fascio-cutaneous flap and as a fascio-myocutaneous chimeric flap consisting of the fascia and a portion of the medial gastrocnemius muscle supplied by 2 different perforators arising from the main sural artery to reconstruct the tongue and floor of the mouth. The major benefit of this flap for tongue reconstruction—it is a thin flap and places the donor site in a far less conspicuous area than the radial forearm. Furthermore, the availability of local muscle from the same arterial system enhances its usefulness for floor-of-the-mouth reconstructions. One of its major drawbacks is the tedious nature of the dissection and difficulty of finding a reliable perforator preoperatively to enable successful microvascular repair. The authors recommend the use of an endoscope to confirm the size and location of the donor perforator artery suggested by the use of a hand-held doppler. In 1 instance, it was necessary to harvest the flap from the opposite leg. Further study and experience needs to develop, if possible, a more reliable method for preoperative planning to facilitate the harvesting of this flap.

**S. H. Miller, MD, MPH**

*Reference*

1. Cavadas PC, Sans-Giménez-Rico JR, Gutierrez-de la Cámara. The medial sural artery perforator free flap. *Plast Reconstr Surg.* 2001;108:1609-1615.

---

**Analysis of functional results and quality of life following free jejunal flaps for reconstruction after upper aerodigestive neoplastic resection: the St James's experience**
Hanson RP, Chow TK, Feehan E, et al (St James's Hosp, Dublin)
*J Plast Reconstr Aesthetic Surg* 60:577-582, 2007

---

Surgical treatment of hypopharyngeal cancers with extension to the postcricoid region generally requires a circumferential pharyngolaryngoesphagectomy followed by reconstruction of the upper aerodigestive tract.

Many techniques have been described in order to achieve a safe and functional reconstruction. Interposition of the jejunal free flap (JFF) is a well-established technique and is the flap of choice in our unit.

This is a retrospective review of all patients who required a JFF following pharyngolaryngoesphagectomy, over an 9-year period. We studied medical charts, histological reports, and speech and language therapy assessments. Eight of the nine surviving patients completed a quality of life questionnaire. Analysis was carried out on patient demographics, flap survival, patient survival and quality of life, including swallow function and speech restoration.

A total of 23 patients had 24 jejunal free flaps. There were four perioperative deaths. Two flaps failed, and were salvaged with a second JFF in one case and a gastric pull-up in the second. Functioning swallow was established in 74% of patients, with four patients complaining of dysphagia. Speech was restored, using an electrolarynx or Blom Singer valve, in 70% of patients. Most patients required radiotherapy as part of their adjuvant treatment.

In our hands, the JFF for reconstruction following pharyngolaryngoesophageal resection, allows restoration of function following major ablative surgery.

▶ Studies to document quality of life after major surgery, which in many instances is attempted for cure, but frequently ends up in palliation are, in my opinion, a must. The results of QAL studies need to take into account, and attempt to standardize, when the studies are performed. The view of postoperative events through a lens of delayed reflection tends to be a less stark contrast with ones preoperative condition. It would be very interesting to study these patients at several time intervals during the course of their recuperation, both to detect actual changes in their overall condition and their perception of their overall health. It would also be important to document that patient/trusted agent (friend or relative) understanding and perceptions of the preoperative discussions are realistic vis-a-vis likely outcomes and risks.

**S. H. Miller, MD, MPH**

**Economic Factors Affecting Head and Neck Reconstructive Microsurgery: The Surgeons' and Hospital's Perspective**
Deleyiannis FW-B, Porter AC (Univ of Pittsburgh, PA; Philadelphia College of Osteopathic Medicine)
*Plast Reconstr Surg* 120:157-165, 2007

*Background.*—The purpose of this study was to determine the relative financial value of providing the service of free-tissue transfer for head and neck reconstruction from the surgeons' and hospital's perspective.

*Methods.*—Medical and hospital accounting records of 58 consecutive patients undergoing head and neck resections and simultaneous free-flap reconstruction were reviewed. Software from the Center for Medicare and Medicaid Services was used to calculate anticipated Medicare payments to the surgeon, based on current procedural terminology codes and to the hospital based on diagnosis-related group codes.

*Results.*—The mean actual payment to the surgeon for a free flap was $2300.60. This payment was 91.6 percent ($2300 out of $2510) of the calculated payment if all payments had been reimbursed by Medicare. Total charges and total payment to the hospital, for the 58 patients, were $19,148,852 and $2,765,552, respectively. After covering direct costs, total hospital revenue (i.e., margin) was $1,056,886. The most commonly assigned diagnosis-related group code was 482 ($n = 35$). According to the fee schedule for that code, if Medicare had been the insurance plan for these 35 patients, the mean payment to the hospital would have been $45,840. The actual mean hospital payment was $44,133. This actual hospital payment represents 96 percent of the calculated Medicare hospital payment ($44,133 of $45,840).

*Conclusions.*—Free-flap reconstruction of the head and neck generates substantial revenue for the hospital. For their mutual benefit, hospitals should join with physicians in contract negotiations of physician reimbursement with insurance companies. Bolstered reimbursement figures would better attract and retain skilled surgeons dedicated to microvascular reconstruction.

▶ Studies, such as these, are very important if we are to have data to document what many surgeons performing lengthy complex procedures seem to know; physician/surgeon reimbursement is too low to justify continuing to perform these complex procedures. Were one to initiate a similar study showing the net loss, based on opportunity costs to the physician, this point would be made even more clearly.

The authors make a valid point about the potential economic loss to large institutions, should physicians choose not to perform these operations.

Although one solution is for physicians to join hospitals in renegotiating reimbursement, there are several potential unintended consequences, which might come from in effect, becoming a "contract employee" of a large institution for one type of operation. However, of greater concern, to me, is the failure to honor our professional commitment to patients to provide the very best, and most appropriate, medical and surgical care. Furthermore, the dictates of professionalism suggest that it is our obligation to bring this issue to those most affected, our patients, and the health plans which profess great concern for quality, rather than just cost factors.

**S. H. Miller, MD, MPH**

---

**Optimal Use of Microvascular Free Flaps, Cartilage Grafts, and a Paramedian Forehead Flap for Aesthetic Reconstruction of the Nose and Adjacent Facial Units**
Burget GC, Walton RL (Univ of Chicago)
*Plast Reconstr Surg* 120:1171-1207, 2007

---

*Background.*—Facial reconstruction with only free microvascular flaps has rarely produced an aesthetic result. Menick stated, "Distant skin always appears as a mismatched patch within residual normal facial skin." In addition, earlier techniques using a single large nasal lining flap or bilateral nasal lining vaults incurred a high incidence of airway obstruction.

*Methods.*—The authors describe 10 consecutive patients requiring reconstruction of the nasal vestibule and columella lining from October of 1997 through May of 2005. Most of them also required reconstruction of the floor of the nose, the platform on which the alar bases and columella rest, and defects of the facial units adjacent to the nose. Aesthetic nasal reconstruction used two separate skin paddles to reconstruct the lining for the nasal vestibule and columella, an artistically constructed nasal framework made of cartilage, a forehead flap for cover, and other flaps and grafts to reconstruct adjacent facial unit defects.

*Results.*—The average patient age was 41.8 years (range, 10.4 to 65.3 years). Follow-up (from the time of the first operative stage) averaged 26.4 months (range, 4 to 49 months). Nine patients had functional airways, and one required nasal airway support with internal silicone tubes. At the time of publication, eight patients had normal-appearing noses, and two were awaiting secondary surgery to correct persistent deformity.

*Conclusions.*—Microvascular free flaps have proved to be highly reliable and efficacious for restoration of missing elements of the nasal lining and adjacent facial soft-tissue defects in total and subtotal nasal reconstruction. Combined with a forehead flap, this aesthetic approach allows for reconstruction of the center of the face layer by layer and facial unit

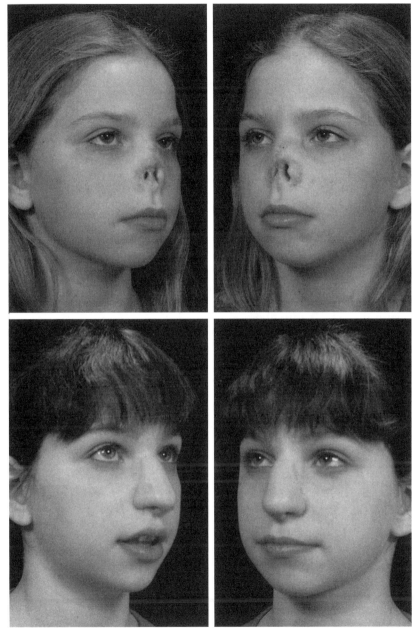

FIGURE 15.—Case 2. Additional preoperative (*above*) and postoperative (*below*) views of the patient. (Reprinted from Burget GC, Walton RL. Optimal use of microvascular free flaps, cartilage grafts, and a paramedian forehead flap for aesthetic reconstruction of the nose and adjacent facial units. *Plast Reconstr Surg.* 2007;120:1171-1207, with permission from the American Society of Plastic Surgeons.)

by facial unit. Specific attention is paid to the artistic creation of normal nasal dimensions, proportion, and form using carved and assembled cartilage grafts and by secondary subcutaneous contouring. In addition, this technique produces a patent airway (Fig 15).

▶ It's hard to argue with 2 surgical giants reporting spectacular results, so I'll say a little more than that this is a "must read" for anyone attempting complex multi layer nose reconstruction. They have set a spectacular standard; it will be hard for the rest of us to match them.

**W. L. Garner, MD**

## Analysis of Salvage Treatments following the Failure of Free Flap Transfer Caused by Vascular Thrombosis in Reconstruction for Head and Neck Cancer

Okazaki M, Asato H, Takushima A, et al (Univ of Tokyo; Kyorin Univ, Mitaka, Japan; Saitama Med School, Moroyama, Japan; et al)
*Plast Reconstr Surg* 119:1223-1232, 2007

*Background.*—Few authors have reported the subsequent treatment for patients in whom free tissue transfers in the head and neck have failed, as a result of vascular thrombosis.

*Methods.*—Between 1993 and May of 2005, 502 free flaps were transferred after head and neck cancer ablation in the authors' hospital, 19 of which resulted in total necrosis caused by vascular thrombosis. The authors categorized these 19 cases into four groups and analyzed the salvage treatment.

*Results.*—For failed free jejunal transfer, early initiation of oral intake was obtained when another free jejunum was transferred. For failed free soft-tissue transfer for intraoral defects, reconstruction with common free (first choice) or pedicled flaps was used: a voluminous musculocutaneous flap for extensive defects, forearm flap or pedicled pectoralis major flap for intermediate defects, and direct closure for small defects of the oral floor. For failed secondary soft-tissue transfer to improve a certain function, salvage flap transfer was not chosen in the acute setting. For failed secondary maxillary reconstruction, simple reconstruction using the rectus abdominis musculocutaneous flap, combined with costal cartilage, achieved stable results. The overall success rate of the repeated free flap was 89 percent (eight of nine patients).

*Conclusions.*—When a free flap is judged unsalvageable, surgeons should determine subsequent treatments, considering the success rate as one of the most important factors. The authors believe that simple reconstruction using a common free flap is the first choice in most cases. When regional or general conditions do not permit further free flap transfer, or when defects are comparatively small, reconstruction with a pedicled flap or direct closure of the defect may be considered.

▶ These author's present their experience in dealing with failed free flaps after reconstruction in the head and neck. In their extensive experience of reconstruction of head and neck defects (502 free flaps), after resections for cancer, failures occurred in 19% or 3.8% of the total. The present study concentrates on these failures and subsequent treatment. Failures were arbitrarily grouped into 4 groups, according to the reason for the primary reconstruction and the subsequent course and therapy for each, outlined in some detail. The options for secondary reconstruction are then detailed and include a second free flap-success rate of 89%. Secondary reconstructions were performed with a new free flap, with a pedicle flap if local conditions preclude a second free flap and if the defects are small, direct closure. This is a valuable report, worthy of careful study by those responsible for reconstruction of major head and neck defects.

**S. H. Miller, MD, MPH**

---

**Postoperative Medical Complications—Not Microsurgical Complications—Negatively Influence the Morbidity, Mortality, and True Costs after Microsurgical Reconstruction for Head and Neck Cancer**
Jones NF, Jarrahy R, Song JI, et al (Univ of California Los Angeles)
*Plast Reconstr Surg* 119:2053-2060, 2007

---

*Background.*—Immediate reconstruction of composite head and neck defects using free tissue transfer is an accepted treatment standard. There remains, however, ongoing debate on whether the costs associated with this reconstructive approach merit its selection, especially considering poor patient prognoses and the high cost of care.

*Methods.*—A retrospective review of the last 100 consecutive patients undergoing microsurgical reconstruction for head and neck cancer by the two senior surgeons was performed to determine whether microsurgical complications or postoperative medical complications had the more profound influence on morbidity and mortality outcomes and the true costs of these reconstructions.

*Results.*—Two patients required re-exploration of the microsurgical anastomoses, for a re-exploration rate of 2 percent, and one flap failed, for a flap success rate of 99 percent. The major surgical complication rate requiring a second operative procedure was 6 percent. Sixteen percent had minor surgical complications related to the donor site. Major medical complications, defined as a significant risk to the patient's life, occurred in 5 percent of the patients, but there was a 37 percent incidence of "minor" medical complications primarily caused by pulmonary problems and alcohol withdrawal. Postsurgical complications almost doubled the average hospital stay from 13.5 days for those patients without complications to 24 days for patients with complications. Thirty-six percent of the true cost of microsurgical reconstruction of head and neck cancer was due to the intensive care unit and hospital room costs, and 24 percent was due to operating room costs. Postsurgical complications resulted in a 70.7 percent increase in true costs, reflecting a prolonged stay in the intensive care unit and not an increase in operating room costs or regular hospital room costs.

*Conclusion.*—Postoperative medical complications in these elderly, debilitated patients related to pulmonary problems and alcohol withdrawal were statistically far more important in negatively affecting the outcomes and true costs of microsurgical reconstruction.

▶ This article emphasizes 2 important points—(1) how reliable and sophisticated microvascular reconstruction of the head and neck has become and (2) how important it is to remember that we are taking care of the entire patient, not just a single anatomic unit. The medical complications, 5% major and 37% minor, dwarfed the surgical complications and skyrocketed costs. This group obviously has a cohesive team caring for these patients. It will be interesting to see how their protocol and algorithms combat these medical problems. It would seem that alcohol withdrawal would be easier to combat compared with the pulmonary problems. In either case, improvements must be made to decrease the comorbidities.

**D. J. Smith., Jr, MD**

# Trunk and Perineal Reconstruction

### Choice of flap for the management of deep sternal wound infection – an anatomical classification

Greig AVH, Geh JLC, Khanduja V, et al (Barts and The London NHS Trust)
*J Plast Reconstr Aesthetic Surg* 60:372-378, 2007

*Background.*—Infection of a median sternotomy wound is a rare, albeit, potentially fatal complication because of the risk of mediastinitis and deep sternal wound infection. Current treatment of deep sternal wound infection comprises antibiotics, debridement, and transposition of muscle or omental flaps to fill the anterior mediastinal dead space.

*Methods.*—A retrospective analysis of the deep sternal wound infections treated in our unit, over a nine-year period, was performed.

*Results.*—Out of the 11,903 consecutive coronary artery bypass graft procedures performed, 27 patients were referred to plastic surgery for management of deep sternal wound infection with flaps. Wounds were classified based on their location on the sternum as type A (upper 1/2), B (lower 1/2) or C (whole of sternum). Five patients had type A wounds, 12 type B wounds and 10 type C wounds. The mean age was 68 years and the M:F ratio was 20:7.

TABLE 1.—Classification of Sternal Wounds According to Anatomical Site

| Wound Type | Site of Sternal Wound | No. of Patients | Recommended Flap for Reconstruction |
| --- | --- | --- | --- |
| Type A | Upper half sternum | 5 (19%) | Pectoralis major |
| Type B | Lower half sternum | 12 (44%) | Combined pectoralis major and rectus abdominis bipedicled flap |
| Type C | Whole sternum | 10 (37%) | Combined pectoralis major and rectus abdominis bipedicled flap |

(Courtesy of Greig AVH, Geh JLC, Khanduja V, et al. Choice of flap for the management of deep sternal wound infection – an anatomical classification. *J Plast Reconstr Aesthetic Surg* 60:372-378, 2007. Reprinted with permission from British Association of plastic, Reconstructive and Aesthetic Surgeon.)

We describe guidelines for the choice of flap for sternal wound reconstruction, according to the anatomical site of the wound dehiscence (Table 1).

▶ The recommendations for flap choice, based on site of wound, are logical and appropriate (maybe some would even consider these obvious). It is, clearly, easier to use just the pectoralis muscle, but this approach works best for upper defects only (see Table 1), and the most sternal wound cases include the lower portion, also (in this series, less than 20% of the cases were exclusively upper sternal wounds). One aspect that is not clear from this report, is whether unilateral or bilateral flaps were used. In my experience, the defect usually requires flaps from both sides to cover the wound and obliterate dead space.

**R. L. Ruberg, MD**

## The Pectoralis Major Muscle Extended Island Flap for Complete Obliteration of the Median Sternotomy Wound
Hallock GG (Lehigh Valley Hospitals and Sacred Heart Hosp, Allentown, PA)
*Ann Plast Surg* 59:655-658, 2007

The sequence of adverse events initiated by a sternal wound infection today can typically be ameliorated by interposing a vascularized flap. The pectoralis major muscle due to its propinquity has universally been the workhorse flap for minimizing this dilemma, with our experience over the past 25 years being no exception as 123 of 156 patients so inflicted required this donor site in some format. However, a rectus abdominis muscle had to be used in combination in 22 patients, particularly for coverage of the xiphoid region, and this can add significant morbidity in an already compromised patient population. This conundrum provided the impetus starting in 2003 for the development of a pectoralis major muscle extended island flap, whereby skeletonizing its vascular pedicle back to near the origin of the thoracoacromial axis, the desired extended reach can be obtained. Since that time, 18 pectoralis major muscle extended island flaps have been successfully used, with only a single wound complication still requiring use of a rectus abdominis muscle flap. This has proven to be a reliable option that alone allows complete closure of the median sternotomy wound while avoiding the need for combined flaps with preservation of the rectus abdominis muscle.

▶ The author documents the effectiveness of a single flap for coverage of the full length of sternotomy wounds. He suggests that the use of a single flap may save time (when compared with bilateral flaps), and he cites circumstances in which use of one of the 2 pectoralis muscles is obviated because of previous surgery and/or radiation. But in most situations, both pectoralis muscles *can* be used (even if 1 internal mammary artery has been "borrowed" for coronary revasculaziation). My personal choice is to avoid use of the rectus abdominis muscle (because of donor site concerns), but to use both pectoralis muscles (1 based laterally, 1 based medially) rotated in such a way as to cover virtually all of the sternal defect. The dissection of a medially based pectoralis is usually done quite quickly. If faced with a circumstance in which incomplete coverage will clearly be the result, I now would extend the dissection of my laterally based pectoralis flap (as described by this author), rather than going to the abdomen to harvest the rectus abdominis, to complete the inferior closure.

**R. L. Ruberg, MD**

---

**Intercostal Artery–Based Rectus Abdominis Transposition Flap for Sternal Wound Reconstruction: Fifteen-Year Experience and Literature Review**
Jacobs B, Ghersi MM (Mount Sinai Med Ctr, Miami Beach, FL)
*Ann Plast Surg* 60:410-415, 2008

---

The rectus abdominis transposition (RAT) flap is a well-accepted alternative to pectoralis muscle flaps for sternal reconstruction after debridement in poststernotomy mediastinitis. Use of this flap based on an intercostal artery pedicle, after division of the ipsilateral internal mammary artery (IMA), is a less-recognized option for reconstruction, given its less substantial vascular supply. The authors present 15 cases where intercostal artery–based RAT flaps were used for sternal reconstruction over a span of 15 years. They describe patient demographic data, management approaches, surgical techniques, and clinical outcomes. Perioperative flap survival and wound healing was optimal in all cases. One morbidity and 1 mortality were encountered in patients with multiple chronic medical problems. Follow-up demonstrated optimal surgical results and satisfied patients. Our observations suggest that the intercostal artery–based RAT flap is a safe treatment option for sternal reconstruction when pectoralis muscle flaps have failed or do not adequately provide coverage of sternal defects after debridement of the poststernotomy wound.

▶ The technique, described by these authors, provides a useful addition to our armamentarium of techniques available for sternal wound reconstruction. This is not really a new technique—the use of the intercostal artery blood supply, for perfusion and transfer of the rectus abdominis muscle, has been documented in the past. However, this study now shows that this approach can be effectively, and consistently, applied to the difficult sternal wound. I, personally, prefer pectoralis major flaps (based either medially or laterally, depending on the integrity of the internal mammary artery [IMA]) for coverage of sternal wounds, but in some cases, adequate coverage of the lower portion of the sternum is problematic. The rectus abdominis muscle could provide added coverage to the inferior portion of the sternotomy wound. Now, we know that the rectus abdominis can be used effectively, even if the IMA has been "borrowed" for perfusion of the coronary system.

**R. L. Ruberg, MD**

---

**Reconstruction of complex chest wall defects by using polypropylene mesh and a pedicled latissimus dorsi flap: a 6-year experience**
Hameed A, Akhtar S, Naqvi A, et al (Federal Postgraduate Med Inst, Lahore, Pakistan)
*J Plast Reconstr Aesthetic Surg* 61:628-635, 2008

---

*Background.*—Reconstruction of full thickness defects of the chest wall is controversial and presents a complicated treatment scenario for thoracic and reconstructive plastic surgeons. It requires close cooperation between the cardiothoracic and reconstructive surgeons to achieve an optimal outcome and reduce the incidence of complications.

*Objective.*—The purpose of this study is to evaluate our results in patients who underwent prosthetic bony reconstruction with polypropylene mesh and pedicle latissimus dorsi flap after chest wall resection. The principles of chest wall reconstruction include: wide excision of primary chest wall tumour with macroscopically healthy margins, wound excision and debridement of necrotic devitalised and irradiated tissues, control of infection and local wound care.

*Study Design.*—This is a descriptive study. It includes 20 patients who underwent chest wall resection due to various causes and followed by reconstruction with polypropylene mesh along with pedicled latissimus dorsi flap.

*Place and Duration of Study.*—The study was conducted at the Department of Plastic and Reconstructive Surgery, Federal Postgraduate Medical Institute, Sheikh Zayed Hospital Lahore, over a period of 6 years from August 1999 to August 2005.

*Patients and Methods.*—This study included 20 patients who underwent chest wall reconstruction using polypropylene mesh and pedicled latissimus dorsi flap from August 1999 to August 2005. Patient demographic data including age, sex, pathological diagnosis, extent and type of resection, size of defect, and outcome were recorded. All patients were followed up in our outpatients department for 1 year.

*Results.*—There was a total of 20 patients, 16 males and four females. The average age was 54 years (range 44–64 years). The indications for resection were primary chest wall tumours in 13 (65%) patients, local recurrence from breast tumours in one (5%) patient, post median sternotomy in three (15%) patients and radionecrosis in three (15%) patients. Ribs along with a part of sternum were resected in 14 (70%) patients, ribs along with clavicle in two (10%) patients and ribs only in four (20%) patients. The average area of chest wall defect after resection was 16.5 × 13 cm. In all patients, skeletal defect was reconstructed with polypropylene mesh. Soft tissue coverage was provided with a pedicled latissimus dorsi flap in all cases. Three patients with a chest wall tumour developed a recurrence within 6 months. Among these three, one patient died within 8 months of follow up due to myocardial infarction.

*Conclusion.*—Chest wall resection and reconstruction with synthetic polypropylene mesh and local muscle flaps can be performed as a safe, effective one-stage surgical procedure for a variety of major chest wall defects (Fig 4 and 6).

▶ The authors present an impressive series of chest wall reconstructive cases. The article is selected not only because of the multiple successful reconstructions but also because of the thorough discussion of the principles and options that are applied to the cases. The authors appropriately emphasize the importance of a coordinated effort by plastic surgeons and thoracic surgeons in these complex cases. They review options for reconstructing the bony defect, and present the rationale for their choice (while acknowledging that other surgeons have employed other materials with success). They provide guidelines

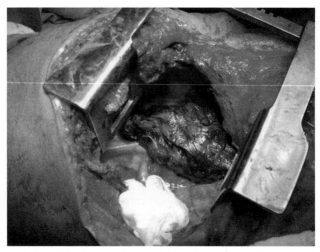

FIGURE 4.—Defect of lateral chest wall after radical excision. (Reprinted from Hameed A, Akhtar S, Naqvi A, et al. Reconstruction of complex chest wall defects by using polypropylene mesh and a pedicled latissimus dorsi flap: a 6-year experience. *J Plast Reconstr Aesthetic Surg.* 2008;61:628-635, with permission from the British Association of Plastic, Reconstructive and Aesthetic Surgeons.)

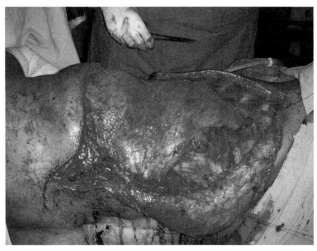

FIGURE 6.—Soft tissue coverage with latissimus dorsi muscle flap from the same side. (Reprinted from Hameed A, Akhtar S, Naqvi A, et al. Reconstruction of complex chest wall defects by using polypropylene mesh and a pedicled latissimus dorsi flap: a 6-year experience. *J Plast Reconstr Aesthetic Surg.* 2008;61:628-635, with permission from the British Association of Plastic, Reconstructive and Aesthetic Surgeons.)

for the size of defects, which warrant (require) substitution for the bony loss, and appropriately differentiate between anterior and posterior chest wounds. Finally, they discuss not only their reasons for choosing this particular flap for coverage (the pedicled latissimus dorsi flap) but also provide information regarding other possible choices when this option is not available in selected cases.

**R. L. Ruberg, MD**

## The Perforator-Sparing Buttock Rotation Flap for Coverage of Pressure Sores
Wong C-H, Tan B-K, Song C (Singapore Gen Hosp)
*Plast Reconstr Surg* 119:1259-1266, 2007

*Background.*—The rotation fasciocutaneous flap for buttock pressure sore coverage has the distinct advantage of allowing rerotation in the event of ulcer recurrence. The authors describe their approach of preserving and incorporating musculocutaneous perforators into the conventional rotation design.

*Methods.*—The skin incision is the same as that for the conventional gluteal rotation flap. The flap is elevated, subfascially, until one or two large musculocutaneous perforators of the superior or inferior gluteal arteries are encountered. Intramuscular dissection by splitting fibers of the gluteus maximus muscle is then performed to free the perforator down to its emergent point at the level of the piriformis muscle to enable the perforator to pivot freely with the rotation of the skin flap. Further elevation of the flap beyond the location of the perforator is then performed, as necessary, to enable tension-free rotation of the skin flap into the defect. Muscle to fill dead space when needed is raised as a separate flap. Seven patients underwent closure of buttock pressure sores in the sacral, ischial, and trochanteric areas using this technique.

*Results.*—All wounds healed, with no recurrence, at a mean follow-up of 30 months. This technique can be used to cover pressure sores over the sacral, trochanteric, and ischial regions.

*Conclusions.*—This modification of the conventional rotation flap affords the flexibility of rerotation in the event of ulcer recurrence, while providing the flap with enhanced blood supply. This is an ideal flap for patients in whom the risk of ulcer recurrence is high.

▶ This article demonstrates application of perforator-preservation techniques to improve the blood supply of a traditional rotation flap. Because this method requires extra time for perforator dissection, I think that it should be used only in highly selected situations. For example, in a paraplegic patient, there is no need to dissect out the perforator because the entire muscle can be rotated without increase in functional impairment. In a patient with normal muscle function, a fasciocutaneous rotation flap without the perforator, usually provides a perfectly viable and durable flap. But in the (rare) situation where the patient has a large ulcer but normal muscle function, this flap should help provide robust tissue and the potential for wide undermining to achieve a successful wound closure.

**R. L. Ruberg, MD**

---

**An Anatomical Study of the Gracilis Muscle and Its Application in Groin Wounds**
Hussey AJ, Laing AJ, Regan PJ (Univ College Hosp, Galway, Ireland)
*Ann Plast Surg* 59:404-409, 2007

---

The management of groin wounds is a common and challenging problem encountered in surgical practice. The purpose of this study is to examine the anatomic basis of the gracilis muscle with relation to this problem. Twelve cadaveric lower limbs were studied to examine both the extramuscular and intramuscular vasculature of the gracilis muscle. These underwent dissection and in 3 cases radiologic examination. The mean entry point of the dominant arterial pedicle was 9.4 cm, with mean length and width of the muscle recorded as 38.4 cm and 6.2 cm, respectively. Each gracilis muscle was then mobilized between the adductor longus and adductor magnus muscles on its dominant pedicle and transposed into the femoral triangle. In each case, the gracilis muscle mobilized easily on its dominant pedicle to adequately cover the groin.

The gracilis muscle is a reliable muscle flap with a consistent blood supply, which can be transposed easily into the groin, based on its dominant pedicle, and offers adequate coverage of the femoral vessels.

▶ A common problem facing plastic surgeons is closure of an open groin wound. In our practice, this problem often involves exposed critical structures following vascular surgery, and the usual solution is rotation of a portion of the sartorius muscle. The proximity of the sartorius makes it a logical and simple choice, but its vascular supply (segmental in nature) can be problematic. I have used the gracilis muscle for a variety of reconstructive problems, but not this one. The advantages of the gracilis for groin wounds would be a more reliable blood supply and a larger potential area of coverage. The disadvantage is that the dissection required to move this muscle into the groin is more extensive than necessary for most other uses of this muscle, and therefore more time consuming. The authors have not given us any clinical evidence of successful use of the gracilis in these cases, only the theoretical basis for its potential use. A follow-up clinical study would be welcomed.

**R. L. Ruberg, MD**

---

**Unilateral gracilis myofasciocutaneous advancement flap for single stage reconstruction of scrotal and perineal defects**
Hsu H, Lin CM, Sun T-B, et al (Buddhist Tzi Chi Gen Hosp, Hualien, Taiwan; Buddhist Dalin Tzi Chi Gen Hosp, Chiayi, Taiwan)
*J Plast Reconstr Aesthetic Surg* 60:1055-1059, 2007

---

*Background.*—Extensive defects of the perineal area, with exposure of the testes, are difficult to reconstruct. Numerous reconstruction methods are available, but few provide us with an aesthetically acceptable, thin and pliable cover. The gracilis myocutaneous flap had the disadvantage of an unreliable skin paddle since McCraw's original description. Our method of using a longitudinally orientated gracilis myofasciocutaneous flap with wide incorporation of the perigracilis fascia, provided us a large reliable cutaneous territory and allowed us to repair extensive perineal defects in one single operation.

*Methods.*—Eight patients treated for Fournier's gangrene between 2003 and 2005 were enrolled in the study. All patients underwent early, aggressive surgical debridement followed by surgical reconstruction with a gracilis myofasciocutaneous flap.

*Results.*—The size of the defect ranged from 12 cm × 7 cm to 30 cm × 15 cm. Diverting colostomy was performed in six of the eight patients. All patients recuperated well with good coverage of the defects. No wound dehiscence due to excessive tension was seen. Haematoma developed in one patient. One patient developed an abscess in the distal part of the donor thigh three months after the initial flap coverage.

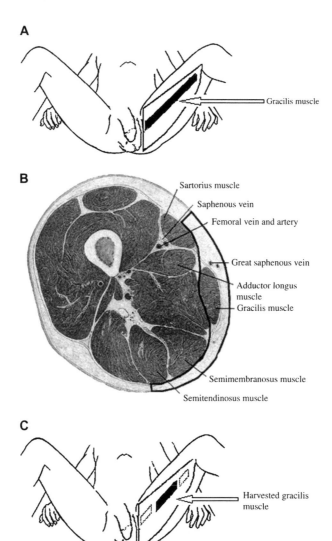

FIGURE 1.—Graphic illustration to demonstrate the design of the flap. (A) The patient is placed in the lithotomy position with the myofasciocutaneous flap designed as a V–Y flap based on the gracilis muscle. The open end of the V is adjacent to the defect and the narrow end is placed distally at the knee. (B) A cross-sectional view of the gracilis muscle at the mid-thigh region demonstrating the dissection plane, with incorporation of the perigracilis fascia. (C) The myofasciocutaneous flap is elevated with the proximal part of the flap elevated without the muscle portion. The distal portion of the gracilis muscle is transected to allow further forward advancement of the flap. (Reprinted from Hsu H, Lin CM, Sun T-B, et al. Unilateral gracilis myofasciocutaneous advancement flap for single stage reconstruction of scrotal and perineal defects. *J Plast Reconstr Aesthetic Surg.* 2007;60:1055–1059. Copyright 2007, with permission from the British Association of Plastic, Reconstructive and Aesthetic Surgeons.)

*Conclusion.*—Gracilis myofasciocutaneous advancement flap provides a good cover for the perineal defect with testicular exposure. It is technically easy and has favourable functional and aesthetic results. It allows the surgeon the ability to reconstruct the perineal and scrotal defects in one single stage (Fig 1).

▶ I have used the gracilis muscle in a variety of ways for reconstructive purposes, but never as a V-Y advancement flap as described by these authors. The muscle is usually a reliable, adequately vascularized structure; the musculocutaneous flap is less reliable. It seems to me that the viability of the skin overlying the muscle is always questionable, and rotating the flap around its vascular pedicle compromises the blood supply even further. So this simple advancement, done leaving the central portion of the muscle attached to its blood supply and unrotated, makes sense. The authors report successful application of this technique in 8 male patients, most of whom had additional, compromising medical conditions. I don't see any reason why this wouldn't be applicable in female patients (eg, for vulvar reconstruction) as well.

**R. L. Ruberg, MD**

---

### Preliminary Experience in Reconstruction of the Vulva Using the Pedicled Vertical Deep Inferior Epigastric Perforator Flap

Santanelli F, Paolini G, Renzi L, et al (Univ of Rome "La Sapienza")
*Plast Reconstr Surg* 120:182-186, 2007

---

*Background.*—Reconstruction of the vulvar area is particularly challenging. Traditionally, bilateral local flaps are required, making closure of the donor area impossible and prolonging the procedure. For very large defects, even bilateral flaps can be insufficient. A procedure for repairing very large vulvar defects after extensive resection was developed that is based on use of a single skin island flap, does not include muscle transfer, and uses a distant donor site.

*Methods.*—Three vulvar reconstructions were done using the vertical deep inferior epigastric perforator (DIEP) flap. The patients included an obese 50-year-old woman whose stage III vulvar squamous cell carcinoma extended to the vaginal introitus; a 62-year-old woman whose stage III squamous cell carcinoma of the vulva and distal third of the vagina required wide tumor excision; and an obese 65-year-old woman who had recurrent vulvar Paget's disease of the vaginal introitus and anus. The procedure begins with the patient in the Lloyd-Davies position and the urinary bladder catheterized. A separate team performs the ablative surgery, with the flap raised vertically from the abdominal wall overlying the rectus abdominis muscle. The flap includes one or more deep inferior epigastric perforators and the umbilicus, which is placed when insetting around the urethral cuff is required. Dissection extends from cranial to caudad in a suprafascial plane. All the epigastric perforators are preserved at first, then 1 or 2 are spared, depending on position and size, and prepared through the rectus muscle. The deep inferior epigastric vessels are dissected to their origin from the iliac artery and vein. After isolating the flap on a long pedicle with a wide arc of rotation, the surgeon places it subcutaneously into the defect. The donor area is then closed in multiple layers after a suction drain is placed. A tunnel remains for the vascular pedicle. This pedicle is placed as low as possible and sutured gently to the muscular fascial layer of the abdominal wall, thereby avoiding kinking of the pedicle. Herniation is still possible. The lateral margin of the flap is sutured to the defect border, whereas the medial margin is sutured to itself and to the proximal vaginal stump. The urethra is then sutured with multiple intercalated flaps to the umbilicus. The patient is allowed to control her analgesia for 3 to 5 days postoperatively and instructed not to adduct the thighs for 1 week, although she can sit. Beginning 8 days after surgery, the patient can ambulate and is discharged 9 days after the procedure.

*Results.*—None of the flaps were totally lost, and all but one healed without incident. The patient with Paget's disease had the longest flap and developed distal tip necrosis requiring debridement. Subsequent healing was uneventful. The donor area healed without complication in all 3 patients. Each woman achieved a symmetrical result with a patent vagina and continent anus.

*Conclusions.*—The vertical DIEP flap proved successful in these extensive vulvar reconstructions. The only complication was a distal 2- to 3-cm necrosis of a 37 × 11-cm flap.

▶ The real value of this technique is the size of the skin paddle that can be achieved with a single flap. When I have had to cover large vulvar defects in the past, I usually have needed 2 flaps (most commonly, gracilis flaps), and therefore, 2 donor sites. This method appears to be more reliable than previous techniques, has minimal functional impairment (no muscle is "sacrificed"), and also facilitates simultaneous closure of the donor and recipient sites. A final "bonus" of this flap is the ability to use the umbilicus to reconstruct the distal urethra!

**R. L. Ruberg, MD**

---

**New Technique of Total Phalloplasty With Reinnervated Latissimus Dorsi Myocutaneous Free Flap in Female-to-Male Transsexuals**
Vesely J, Hyza P, Ranno R, et al (Masaryk Univ in Brno, Czech Republic; Univ of Catania, Italy)
*Ann Plast Surg* 58:544-550, 2007

---

From December 2001 to September 2005, the technique of total penile reconstruction, with a reinnervated free latissimus dorsi myocutaneous flap, was used in 22 patients (24-38 years old) with gender dysphoria.

These patients were followed up for at least 11 months (range, 11-44 months). All flaps survived. Complications include hematoma (7 cases), vascular thrombosis (2 cases), partial necrosis (1 case), excessive swelling of the neophallus (3 cases), and skin graft loss at the donor site (1 case). Of the 19 patients included in the final evaluation, the transplanted muscle was able to obtain contraction in 18 (95%) cases, and 8 patients (42%) had sexual intercourse by contracting the muscle to stiffen and move the neopenis. The described technique of neophalloplasty proved to be a reliable technique, and the muscle movement in the neophallus can be expected in almost all cases. The muscle contraction in the neophallus leads to "paradox" erection—stiffening, widening, and shortening of the neopenis, which allows for sexual intercourse in some patients. Subsequent reconstruction of the urethra is possible.

▶ The aesthetic results, shown in this article, are certainly acceptable (see figure). The functional benefit of using the contraction of the latissimus muscle for intercourse is of questionable value. I think that the choice of technique for total penile reconstruction boils down to one major consideration: How important is it for the patient to have a hidden donor site? If a concealed donor site is of great importance, then this flap (the LD) is probably more suitable than the previous "gold standard" for penile reconstruction: the radial artery forearm flap.

**R. L. Ruberg, MD**

---

**Genital Sensitivity After Sex Reassignment Surgery in Transsexual Patients**
Selvaggi G, Monstrey S, Ceulemans P, et al (Ghent Univ Hosp, Belgium)
*Ann Plast Surg* 58:427-433, 2007

---

*Background.*—Tactile and erogenous sensitivity in reconstructed genitals is one of the goals in sex reassignment surgery. Since November 1993 until April 2003, a total of 105 phalloplasties, with the radial forearm free flap, and 127 vaginoclitoridoplasties, with the inverted penoscrotal skin flap and the dorsal glans pedicled flap, have been performed at Ghent University Hospital. The specific surgical tricks used to preserve genital and tactile sensitivity are presented.

In phalloplasty, the dorsal hood of the clitoris is incorporated into the neoscrotum; the clitoris is transposed, buried, and fixed directly below the reconstructed phallic shaft; and the medial and lateral antebrachial nerves are coapted to the inguinal nerve and to one of the 2 dorsal nerves of the clitoris. In vaginoplasty, the clitoris is reconstructed from a part of the glans penis inclusive of a part of the corona, the inner side of the prepuce is used to reconstruct the labia minora, and the penile shaft is inverted to line the vaginal cavity.

*Material and Methods.*—A long-term sensitivity evaluation (performed by the Semmes-Weinstein monofilament and the Vibration tests) of 27 reconstructed phalli and 30 clitorises has been performed.

*Results.*—The average pressure and vibratory thresholds values for the phallus tip were, respectively, 11.1 g/mm$^2$ and 3 μm. These values have been compared with the ones of the forearm (donor site). The average pressure and vibratory thresholds values for the clitoris were, respectively, 11.1 g/mm$^2$ and 0.5 μm. These values have been compared with the ones of the normal male glans, taken from the literature.

We also asked the examined patients if they experienced orgasm after surgery, during any sexual practice (ie, we considered only patients who attempted to have orgasm): all female-to-male and 85% of the male-to-female patients reported orgasm.

*Conclusion.*—With our techniques, the reconstructed genitalia obtain tactile and erogenous sensitivity. To obtain a good tactile sensitivity in the reconstructed phallus, we believe that the coaptation of the cutaneous nerves of the flap with the ilioinguinalis nerve and with one of the 2 nerves of the clitoris is essential in obtaining this result. To obtain orgasm after phalloplasty, we believe that preservation of the clitoris beneath the reconstructed phallus and some preservation of the clitoris hood are essential. To obtain orgasm after a vaginoplasty, the reconstruction of the clitoris from the neurovascular pedicled glans flap is essential.

▶ This article clearly demonstrates that sex reassignment surgery has passed from the phase of achieving a satisfactory aesthetic result to one of improving function. Also impressive, is that these investigators have performed sex reassignment in more than 230 patients. The article documents the various surgical steps, which these surgeons have developed and refined, in the effort to achieve genital sensitivity. The reader is referred to the "Surgical Technique" section of the article for more specific detail.

**R. L. Ruberg, MD**

# 3 Trauma

## Head, Neck, and Extremity

### A Financial Analysis of Operative Facial Fracture Management

Erdmann D, Price K, Reed S, et al (Private Diagnostic Clinic, Duke Univ Med Ctr, Durham, NC)
*Plast Reconstr Surg* 121:1323-1327, 2008

*Background.*—The financial impact of operative facial fracture management has not been systematically investigated. This study aims to provide a descriptive financial analysis of patients undergoing operative facial fracture management at a single academic medical center and the financial impact on the health system.

*Methods.*—The records of 202 patients who underwent operative facial fracture management over a 3-year period (2003 to 2005) were analyzed. All physician (professional) and hospital charges related to fracture management were included. Professional charges were subdivided by specialty and by payer type; hospital charges included operating room, recovery room, intensive care unit, hospital bed, supply charges, pharmaceuticals, laboratory charges, and radiographs. For comparison, similar data were obtained for the general plastic surgery population and for orthopedic surgery patients.

*Results.*—The sum of all professional charges billed was $2,478,234 (average, $12,268 per patient). Collections for these professional services totaled $675,434, yielding an overall reimbursement rate of 27 percent. Reimbursement rates ranged from 38 percent for critical care physicians to 24 percent for surgery and neuroradiology. The highest collection rates occurred in children covered by the State Children's Health Insurance Program and in prison inmates (53 percent and 99 percent, respectively). The lowest collection rates were obtained from uninsured patients (10 percent total billing over collections). Total hospital charges were $18,120,027 (average, $89,703 per patient); the total collections were $2,770,115 (15 percent reimbursement rate).

*Conclusions.*—This study provides a descriptive financial analysis of operative facial fracture management. The unfavorable financial circumstances associated with facial trauma care may present a challenge to academic medical centers and plastic surgeons.

▶ This is a very interesting article, but I am unsure of how to interpret it for several reasons. First, it is not likely to be generalizable coming from a single center. Second, the problem of charges versus costs has been raised by the authors, but not really answered. The fact that reimbursement levels vary for different providers is a well-recognized phenomenon and based on many factors, not the least of which are the contracts established by the providers and the different payers. Another major problem with this study is that it compares reimbursement percentages for facial fracture patients with total plastic surgical and orthopedic surgical patient populations yet does not provide us with comparable data regarding payer mix in the latter 2 groups. There is little doubt that university and not-for-profit hospitals, especially that associate with providing care to indigents population, are the major safety net for trauma patients in the United States. Furthermore, these institutions, by their very nature and their missions, are more costly to run than are most for-profit hospitals. That being said, if they are to continue to provide the services they do and to operate as safety nets, they need to make a more compelling and generalizable case for higher reimbursement or supplemental funding. This is an excellent area for a multicenter collaborative study, guided in part by 1 or several business schools associated with the University Hospitals participating.

**S. H. Miller, MD, MPH**

---

### The White-Eyed Medial Blowout Fracture
Tse R, Allen L, Matic D (Univ of Western Ontario, London, Canada)
*Plast Reconstr Surg* 119:277-286, 2007

---

*Background.*—The pediatric white-eyed blowout fracture, with entrapment of the inferior rectus muscle, is well recognized as an easily missed injury with significant morbidity if left untreated. A series of five isolated medial orbital blowout fractures, with medial rectus muscle entrapment, is described. The purpose of this study was to define this injury pattern and its clinical outcome.

*Methods.*—A retrospective review of the presentation, management, and clinical outcomes of identified cases was conducted.

*Results.*—Early exploration and release of the entrapped muscle, combined with implant reconstruction of the medial orbital wall, within 2 weeks, resulted in complete resolution of diplopia and full recovery of extraocular movements. Delayed treatment and release of the soft tissues without orbital wall reconstruction, were associated with restricted gaze and diplopia. Similar outcomes were confirmed on analysis of other reported cases.

*Conclusions.*—Orbital floor blowout fractures in the pediatric population have a high incidence of muscle entrapment that must be recognized and treated early to avoid muscle necrosis and permanent ocular restriction from fibrosis. Medial orbital wall fractures with entrapment are rare, but early recognition and operative release of the entrapped muscles result in better outcomes.

▶ I have seen only 1 medial wall blowout fracture. Maybe, the fact that only 37 cases have been reported in the literature explains this. However, the fact that these authors found 5 more of their own cases suggests that the incidence may be higher than expected. The principles of management are no different from those for orbital glow fractures with entrapment. The challenge, here, is making the diagnosis not performing the treatment.

**R. L. Ruberg, MD**

## Nasolacrimal Duct Reconstruction With Nasal Mucoperiosteal Flap

Lee J-W (Natl Cheng-Kung Univ Hosp, Tainan, Taiwan, ROC)
*Ann Plast Surg* 59:143-148, 2007

Surgical repair of lacrimal drainage apparatus may be quite difficult in patients with maxillofacial injuries involving extensive structural damage. When the primary tear tract has become nonamendable or inaccessible, it would then be necessary to set up an alternate draining route for tear passage.

Conjunctivorhinostomy with a Jones tube is an effective diversionary treatment method, and yet, this procedure might be plagued with problems related to alloplastic device usage. Autologous tissue is, therefore, best suited for nasolacrimal conduit restoration.

A superiorly based mucoperiosteal flap, 11 to 13 mm in width and 20 to 25 mm in vertical length, is mobilized from lateral nasal wall and fashioned into a tubelike conduit. This construct is then turned superior-laterally and connected to the conjunctival sac. The fistula tract, thus formed, has a sufficiently large caliber and is lined, entirely, with normal mucosal epithelium. Such a feature may exert a favorable influence upon the long-term patency of the tear passage.

This approach is applied, successfully, in 3 consecutive patients of lacrimal system obstruction, one of whom even had experienced 2 failed attempts of Jones tube insertion beforehand. The tactics and experiences in managing these 3 cases form the basis of this report.

▶ The performance of the Jones procedure has become a standard fixture in the armamentarium of surgeons dealing with injuries or destruction of the nasolacrimal duct. Although simple to perform and usually successful in the short-term, long-term postoperative results are not infrequently unsatisfactory for the patient and include recurrent conjunctival irritation, malposition and loss of the Pyrex tube, and the need for lifetime maintenance of the tube. Consequently, several authors have suggested reconstruction of the nasolacrimal apparatus with autologous tissue. This author suggests using a local nasal mucoperisteal flap, from the upper nasal vault, and fashioned into a tube-like conduit, which is connected to the conjunctiva on the affected side. The report only details 3 patients, and although fustulagrams show patency, the longest follow-up fistualgram is 5 months, post operatively, and only in one of the 3 patients. The procedure requires an external facial incision, but this should be well-hidden in the nasal cheek crease, providing the scar heals kindly.

**S. H. Miller, MD, MPH**

---

**Intralesional steroid injection for the management of otohematoma**
Im GJ, Chae SW, Choi J, et al (College of Medicine, Korea Univ, Seoul, South Korea)
*Otolaryngol Head Neck Surg* 139:115-119, 2008

---

*Objectives.*—To compare the therapeutic efficacies of aspiration plus intralesional steroid injection and aspiration plus pressure dressing for the management of otohematoma.

*Study Design and Setting.*—Fifteen patients with otohematoma were treated by aspiration plus pressure dressing (the pressure dressing group) and 34 patients were treated with intralesional steroid injections followed by simple aspiration (the steroid injection group).

*Results.*—Otohematoma resolved within four weeks in all 15 patients in the pressure dressing group, but eight of the 15 showed perichondrial thickening. The duration of treatment was shorter in the steroid injection group than in the pressure dressing group; 14 (41.2%) of the 34 recovered after the first injections and another 15 (44.1%) after the second, and the remaining 5 (14.7%) after the third without any complications. However, multiple steroid injections are needed due to a high early recurrence rate.

*Conclusion.*—Intralesional steroid injection is the treatment of choice for the management of otohematoma. The correction of causative use of a hard pillow, a helmet, and headphones is essential to prevent late recurrence.

▶ The authors purport to show that intra-cavitary steroid injection is the treatment of choice in patients with otohematoma. This hypothesis is by no means a new one, having been discussed by many authors over several years. However, the evidence provided by the authors in this study is not terribly convincing for several reasons: 1) The study is retrospective, 2) The treatment groups were not randomly selected and as a matter of fact the type of treatment was only a function of when the patients were seen (ie, 1997-98 for aspiration and pressure as opposed to aspiration and steroid in the post 1998 years), 3) Patients in the pressure group were few in number and treated with 2 different pressure modalities, and finally 4) The failure to assess whether the ultimate outcome (perichondral thickening and distortion not measured or quantified beyond the use of the term mild thickening in the pressure-treated ears) is significantly more of a problem than the repeated recurrences with steroid treatment. Furthermore, the frequency of use of intralesional steroid in this study (once a week) was likely inadequate. Clearly, resolution of this issue will necessitate a randomized controlled study, and while the authors are doing so one might add an additional arm-intracavitary steroid plus pressure.

**S. H. Miller, MD, MPH**

---

**Mini replants: Fingertip replant distal to the IP or DIP joint**
Dautel G, Barbary S (Hôpital Jeanne d'Arc, Dommartin les Toul, France)
*J Plast Reconstr Aesthetic Surg* 60:811-815, 2007

---

Amputations through the distal interphalangeal joint or distal to this joint are frequent and they represent probably one of the best indications for replantation. Details on the vascular anatomy of the fingertip have to be perfectly known by the surgeon who will have to deal with these replantations. Factors such as age, mechanism of amputation and type of anastomosis will influence the overall success rate of the procedure. Return of a true static two points discrimination can be observed in children even in the absence of any neural repair.

▶ It is interesting to see this article at nearly the same time as we are evaluating the decrease in replantation and microsurgery. It is fitting, I believe, this comes from the unit with historical lineage to Jacques Michon, Michele Merle, and Guy Foucher. Most surprising to me was the statement—"Although the aesthetic outcome of these replantations was not perfect, this was largely compensated for by the functional benefits." No data is provided so I continue to believe that aesthetics improve more than function. No question this is the best tip reconstruction. In the United States, the question is whether the procedure will be undertaken.

**D. J. Smith, Jr, MD**

---

**Rational flap selection and timing for coverage of complex upper extremity trauma**
Herter F, Ninkovic M, Ninkovic M (Klinikum Muenchen-Bogenhausen, Munich; Innsbruck Med Univ, Austria)
*J Plast Reconstr Aesthetic Surg* 60:760-768, 2007

---

Reconstruction of complex extremity trauma continues to be a challenging task for plastic surgeons. Characteristics of such injuries include destruction of functional structures, often due to high energy trauma that causes significant invalidity. Before the era of free flaps, pedicled fasciocutaneous and muscle flaps were the only option for reconstruction of the severely injured upper extremity. The management of complex injuries of the upper extremity has changed with the development of reconstructive microsurgery.

Nowadays, we have a great variety of different free flaps to cover defects of the upper extremity and restore function by innervated free flaps. Sensibility, skin thickness, texture, colour, durability, binding of the flap to the underlying structures, donor site morbidity, possibility of secondary reconstructive procedures, the surgeon's experience and operative facilities must all be taken into consideration for choosing the optimal reconstructive procedure. Not only the reconstructive und functional requirements but the timing of reconstruction is extremely important for final result.

The purpose of this paper is to define the principles of flap selection and timing of flap reconstruction, according to the assessment of trauma in the upper limb.

▶ I thoroughly enjoyed this article because it forced me to analyze my own algorithm for upper extremity wound closure. I agree with the author's premise that in general, using a local muscle or segment of intact skin in an already traumatized extremity should be avoided. The only exception might be the use of the latissimus flap for repair in the upper arm. The author's note, "We are increasingly of the opinion that free tissue transfer provides of the most appropriate repair of most severe injuries of the extremity." Beyond that, the authors discuss the reconstructive, functional, and timing requirements for picking the optimal reconstructive procedure. I didn't agree with all their prioritizations. What is important is for of each plastic surgeon to have worked through his/her own algorithm and be able to apply it for each individual case.

**D. J. Smith, Jr, MD**

---

### Free Functioning Muscle Transfer for Lower Extremity Posttraumatic Composite Structure and Functional Defect

Lin C-H, Lin Y-T, Yeh J-T, et al (Chang Gung Univ, Taipei, Taiwan)
*Plast Reconstr Surg* 119:2118-2126, 2007

---

*Background.*—Traumatized lower extremities may present not only composite soft-tissue defects, but also, flexor and/or extensor loss. Free functioning muscle transfer can provide composite structural and functional restoration.

*Methods.*—From 1996 to 2004, 19 patients with lower extremity injuries whose lesions exhibited composite soft-tissue damage, with or without bone defects, and certain accompanying functional disabilities were allocated to study groups on the basis of impression, as follows: group I, open fracture IIIB $(n = 10)$; group II, neglected compartment syndromes [open IIIB $(n = 4)$ and open IIIC $(n = 1)$]; and group III, crush injuries $(n = 4)$. Free flap resurfacing was indicated for these lesions. Fifteen patients underwent free functioning muscle transfer; source muscles were the rectus femoris $(n = 3)$, rectus femoris with anterolateral thigh flap $(n = 5)$, and gracilis (for ankle dorsiflexion) $(n = 7)$. Two patients underwent composite rectus femoris and vascular iliac crest for ankle dorsiflexion and segmental tibial defect reconstruction. Two received rectus femoris muscle and anterolateral thigh flaps for posterior compartment defect and quadriceps defect reconstruction, individually.

*Results.*—Two patients required reexploration; salvage was successful in only one, with below-knee amputation necessary in the other. Skin grafts were needed for partial skin paddle necrosis $(n = 3)$ or remaining skin defect $(n = 2)$. Functioning muscle reinnervation failed in four cases, with one individual undergoing ankle fusion, two people electing ambulation with stiff ankles, and one person using an orthosis. In the sample population, range of motion varied and was related to the severity of injury and the extent of skin grafting on the distal musculotendinous portion. Less function was exhibited in the compartment syndrome group (group II).

*Conclusion.*—Functioning muscle transfer can be performed posttraumatically in lower limbs with composite soft-tissue and motor-unit defects, resulting in acceptable functional results and reliable limb salvage.

▶ Much has been written about salvage of lower limbs through free tissue transfer, and about functional muscle transfer to other areas of the body. These authors have combined these 2 ideas to show that lower extremities can not only be salvaged, but even restored to function through the use of free muscle transfers. It appears as though many of their cases were circumstances in which the surgeon might have considered amputation because of the severity of the injury; however, the availability of this technique avoided the amputation and provided a very satisfying result. Similar principles can also be applied to surgical restoration of function after major cancer extirpation procedures of the extremities.

**R. L. Ruberg, MD**

---

**The Fate of Lower Extremities With Failed Free Flaps: A Single Institution's Experience Over 25 Years**
Culliford AT IV, Spector J, Blank A, et al (Staten Island Univ Hosp, NY; Weill Cornell Med College, NY; New York Univ Med Ctr, NY)
*Ann Plast Surg* 59:18-22, 2007

---

*Background.*—Lower-extremity reconstruction with microvascular free flap coverage is often the only option for limb salvage. Flap failure rates, however, continue to have higher complication rates than those to other anatomic sites; a significant number of flaps that fail result in amputation. This study retrospectively analyzed patients treated at a single institution who underwent attempted lower-extremity limb salvage with microsurgical techniques over a 25-year period. Of particular interest are the outcome data for patients who had initial free flap failure.

*Patients and Methods.*—A prospectively maintained database was used to identify patients who satisfy criteria. Every patient who was treated with a microvascular free flap to their lower extremities was identified and included in this analysis. All records were reviewed from 1980 through 2004. Patients who had free flaps to the lower extremity fail after the initial operation were identified and selected for further analysis.

*Results.*—Five hundred eighty-eight patients who underwent microsurgical reconstruction of lower extremity wounds had a failure rate of 8.5%. Trauma patients (83%) had a failure rate of 9%. On subset analysis, the failure rate for trauma patients decreased from 11% (1980–1992) to 3.7% (1993–2004). Of patients who had a failed free flap, 18% went on to limb amputation; the remainder was salvaged with secondary free flaps, local flaps, or skin grafting.

*Conclusion.*—This single institutional experience spanning 25 years represents the longest continual series of lower-extremity free flaps reported in the literature. The improved success rate seen in the second half of the study period is attributed to a more critical selection of free-flap candidates, improved understanding of the physiology surrounding acute trauma and a more sophisticated multidisciplinary team organization.

▶ Plastic surgeons are remarkably bad about admitting our failures and their consequences. These authors should be congratulated simply on facing the facts of our imperfection. There are interesting questions from this series. Forty percent of the 50 patients (9%) were free flap failures or skin grafted. If the wounds were skin graftable, why was free flap being used? It brings out the interesting question of the effects of the flap used as a biologic dressing improving the wound bed (some of you would suggest only the vacuum-assisted closure [VAC] could accomplish this). The amputation rate was low and these authors prove that free flap failure should not be taken as a final outcome. Congratulations on an interesting series and the courage and honesty to present it to us.

**W. L. Garner, MD**

---

**Gustilo Grade IIIB Tibial Fractures Requiring Microvascular Free Flaps: External Fixation Versus Intramedullary Rod Fixation**
Rohde C, Greives MR, Cetrulo C, et al (Columbia Univ Med Ctr, NY; Nassau County Med Ctr, East Meadow, NY; New York Univ Med Ctr, NY)
*Ann Plast Surg* 59:14-17, 2007

---

*Background.*—Gustilo IIIB fractures involve high-energy tibial fractures for which there is inadequate soft tissue coverage. In addition to orthopedic fixation, these injuries require soft tissue reconstruction, often in the form of a microvascular free flap. Although the majority of orthopedic literature favorably compares intramedullary rod fixation to external fixation in open tibial fractures, these studies have not focused on the role of either method of fixation in relation to the soft tissue reconstruction.

*Methods.*—Because we had noted numerous complications after providing free-flap coverage over intramedullary rodded fractures, we sought to investigate whether there were differences in outcomes between free flap–covered lower-extremity fractures which were fixated by external fixation versus intramedullary rods. A retrospective chart review was performed on all patients in our institution who had lower-extremity free flaps for coverage of Gustilo IIIB fractures from 1995–2005 in relation to the type of bony fixation.

*Results.*—Of the 38 patients studied, 18 underwent external fixation of the tibial fracture, and 20 had intramedullary rodding. Overall flap survival was 95%, with 1 failure in each group. However, the intramedullary rod group had higher incidences of wound infection, osteomyelitis, and bony nonunion (25%, 25%, and 40%, respectively) than the external fixation group (6%, 11%, 17%, respectively).

*Conclusions.*—For Gustilo IIIB fractures that require free-flap coverage, the added bony and soft tissue manipulation required for intramedullary rodding may disrupt the surrounding blood supply and lead to higher rates of complications that threaten the overall success of the reconstruction. Plastic and orthopedic surgeons should discuss the optimal method of bony fixation for complex tibial fractures when a free flap will likely be needed for soft tissue coverage. This integrated team approach may help minimize complications.

▶ Plastic surgeons are often called to see patients with these problems and accept that wound healing difficulties and failed fracture healing rates are part of the pathophysiology. These authors suggest the situation may not be simple and provide comparative, although not randomized perspective data that these patients should be treated with external fixation. It is an interesting idea that should be subjected to further analysis, but the differences and outcome are compelling. We should be discussing this with our orthopedic colleagues before they call us "to fill the hole."

**W. L. Garner, MD**

# Burns

**Body image, mood and quality of life in young burn survivors**
Pope SJ, Solomons WR, Done DJ, et al (Univ of Hertfordshire, Hatfield, England)
*Burns* 33:747-755, 2007

This study looks at the body image, mood and quality of life of a group of 36 young people aged between 11 and 19 years who had burns as children, compared with an age-matched control group of 41 young people who had not had these injuries. Participants completed the Body Esteem Scale (BES), the Satisfaction With Appearance Scale (SWAP), the Beck

Depression Inventory-II (BDI-II) and the Youth Quality of Life Question-naire (YQOL). It was hypothesised that young burn survivors would report more dissatisfaction with their appearance, a lower mood and a lower quality of life compared with non-injured controls. However, young burn survivors reported significantly more positive evaluations of how others view their appearance ($p = 0.018$), more positive weight satis-faction ($p = 0.001$) and a higher quality of life ($p = 0.005$) than the control group. They also reported more positive general feelings about their appearance, although this was just below the level for statistical signifi-cance ($p = 0.067$) and a similar mood to the school sample ($p = 0.824$). The data suggest that young burn survivors appear to be coping well in comparison to their peers, and in some areas may be coping better, in spite of living with the physical, psychological and social consequences of burns.

▶ This article should be read with another article by Wisely et al.[1] They both originate in the United Kingdom and attempt to approach the psychological problems of the burned patient. Psychological studies are woefully lacking in burned patients when compared with all the other pathophysiology studies in these trauma patients. Their findings in young burn survivors are not surprising because the Galveston Shrine studies have revealed that children with life-threatening burns and severe alteration of body image achieve the same mile-stones as their unburned peers. Approaching the needs of the adult population is extraordinarily difficult because of the frequency of burned adults who come with incredible mental baggage. The incidence of addiction, alcohol, or drugs in those burned while committing illegal acts is significant. The authors are to be commended for at least trying to elucidate some of the problems.

**R. E. Salisbury, MD**

*Reference*

1. Wisely JA, Hoyle E, Tarrier N, Edwards J. Where to start? Attempting to meet the psychological needs of burned patients. *Burns.* 2007;33:736-746.

---

**Toxic epidermal necrolysis (TEN) and Stevens–Johnson syndrome (SJS): Experience with high-dose intravenous immunoglobulins and topical conservative approach: A retrospective analysis**
Stella M, Clemente A, Bollero D, et al (CTO Hosp, Torino, Italy; et al)
*Burns* 33:452-459, 2007

---

Toxic epidermal necrolysis (TEN) and Stevens–Johnson syndrome (SJS) are rare, drug-induced, severe acute exfoliative skin and mucosal disor-ders.

Several treatments previously proposed have produced contradictory results in small series; in 1998 the use of intravenous immunoglobulins (IVIG) was introduced with excellent clinical findings.

Our experience (1999–2005) using IVIG in the therapy of TEN/SJS, together with a local conservative approach, is reported and related to our previous treatments (1993–1998). The SCORTEN and the standardized mortality ratio (SMR) was used to evaluate the efficacy of our therapeutic modalities.

Eight patients were treated before IVIG era and 23 patients have been treated with IVIG. There was no significant difference in SCORTEN between the two groups. Concerning the local approach, a conservative wound management in IVIG series replaced an extensive epidermal debridment and coverage with artificial skin substitutes of the pre-IVIG series. Overall mortality in patients treated before IVIG was 75% (6/8), in the IVIG group it decreased to 26% (6/23) with a cessation of further epidermal detachment after an average of 5 days (3–10 days) from the onset of the therapy. The SMR showed a trend to lower actual mortality (not significant) with IVIG treatment than the predicted mortality (SMR = 0.728; 95% CI: 0.327–1.620).

▶ This article is worth reading because it summarizes many of the problems of treating toxic epidermal necrolysis (TEN) and the bibliography is good. Unfortunately, the authors do not prove that giving immunoglobulin truly helps. The study suffers from the deficiencies of all retrospective analyses. Treatments were changed, there were multiple drugs given, which could have altered the results and, certainly, the treating physicians were not the same. Having considered these facts, we still give IgV because the mortality from a full-blown case of TEN is greater than that of a similar size burn in our center.

**R. E. Salisbury, MD**

---

**Cooling of the burn wound: The ideal temperature of the coolant**
Venter THJ, Karpelowsky JS, Rode H (Univ of Cape Town, South Africa)
*Burns* 33:917-922, 2007

---

*Background.*—The beneficial effects of cooling a fresh burn wound were well demonstrated. However, there are still conflicting reports as to the optimum temperature of coolant, duration of application and effects in limiting tissue damage. A study was undertaken to investigate this, the importance of the temperature of, and the time period of application of the coolant.

*Materials and Methods.*—Four identical deep dermal wounds were created on the back of 10 anaesthetised pigs. Each animal served as an independent experimental model. The effectiveness of cooling was monitored by measuring intradermal temperatures. The animals were divided into two groups; using ice water and tap water as the coolants. In each pig one wound was not cooled (wound 1). Three were cooled; one immediately for 30 min in group 1 and for 4 h in group 2 (wound 2). The other two wounds were cooled after 30 min for 30 min and 3 h (wounds 3 and 4, respectively).

*Results.*—It was found that the temperature of the coolant was crucial. When ice water of 1-8°C (group 1) was used more necrosis than in the wounds that were not cooled was seen. When tap water was used at 12-18°C (group 2) it was demonstrated clinically and histologically that the cooled wounds had less necrosis than the uncooled wounds and thus healed faster. In group 2 the beneficial effects of cooling were still present when delayed for half an hour.

*Conclusion.*—First aid cooling of a burn wound with tap water is an effective method of minimising the damage sustained during a burn, and is universally and immediately available. Ice water cooling is associated with an increase in tissue damage.

▶ This nicely controlled study examines 2 variables, temperature, and time of application of the coolant. The results are interesting but not shocking. The authors note that icing a wound can cause even more necrosis compared with not treating the wound with coolant and recommend tap water for the cooling. In short, delay before treatment was instituted did not seem to be deleterious and the authors recommended treatment for 3 hours after the thermal insult. A nice explanation for these improved results based on the suppression of histamine release, and a good bibliography, make this article helpful.

**R. E. Salisbury, MD**

---

**Tap water scalds among seniors and the elderly: Socio-economics and implications for prevention**
Alden NE, Bessey PQ, Rabbitts A, et al (New York Presbyterian-Weill Cornell Med Ctr, NY; et al)
*Burns* 33:666-669, 2007

---

*Introduction.*—Tap water scalds among those ≥60 years old are often attributed to physical impairments with aging. This study assesses socio-economics associated with tap water scalds among seniors and the elderly.

*Methods.*—Charts of patients admitted to an urban Burn Center between 7/00 and 6/04 for treatment of tap water scalds were reviewed. Demographics, injury details, co-morbidities, surgical interventions/critical care requirements, length of stay (LOS), disposition and related economics were reviewed.

*Results.*—During the study period, 68 patients ≥60 years were hospitalized for treatment of these scalds. Mean age and burn size were 78 ± 1 years and 7 ± 0.9% TBSA. Over 98% of patients were admitted with pre-existing co-morbidities; 60% required ICU care for 40 ± 5 days; 22% required mechanical ventilation and 71% required surgery. LOS was 34 ± 4 days. Most patients received government assistance income. Pre-injury, 32% resided alone. Post-injury, 10% of patients returned home alone; mortality was 22%. Per patient hospital costs approximated $113,000.

*Conclusion.*—These findings report that tap water scalds result in significant morbidity, mortality and health care costs for local seniors and the elderly. Socio-economic factors play a significant role in these injuries and must be assessed when planning prevention efforts.

▶ This article is extremely interesting, highlighting the results from a major burn center providing excellent care for the elderly. The conclusions are embarrassing, in that they underscore the paucity of efforts being made on behalf of the elderly. Although resources for the pediatric population seem infinite, little has been done in solid prevention for the elderly, especially for those of modest means and human support services. These authors beautifully show the results, including the cost, significant morbidity, and mortality.

**R. E. Salisbury, MD**

## The Effects of Preexisting Medical Comorbidities on Mortality and Length of Hospital Stay in Acute Burn Injury: Evidence From a National Sample of 31,338 Adult Patients

Thombs BD, Singh VA, Halonen J, et al (Johns Hopkins Univ School of Medicine, Baltimore, MD; St Agnes Hosp, Baltimore, MD)
*Ann Surg* 245:629-634, 2007

*Objective.*—To determine whether and to what extent preexisting medical comorbidities influence mortality risk and length of hospitalization in patients with acute burn injury.

*Summary Background Data.*—The effects on mortality and length of stay of a number of important medical comorbidities have not been examined in acute burn injury. Existing studies that have investigated the effects of medical comorbidities on outcomes in acute burn injury have produced inconsistent results, chiefly due to the use of relatively small samples from single burn centers.

*Methods.*—Records of 31,338 adults who were admitted with acute burn injury to 70 burn centers from the American Burn Association National Burn Repository, were reviewed. A burn-specific list of medical comorbidities was derived from diagnoses included in the Charlson Index of Comorbidities and the Elixhauser method of comorbidity measurement. Logistic regression was used to assess the effects of preexisting medical conditions on mortality, controlling for demographic and burn injury characteristics. Ordinal least squares regression with a logarithmic transformation of the dependent variable was used to assess the relationship of comorbidities with length of stay.

*Results.*—In-hospital mortality was significantly predicted by HIV/AIDS (odds ratio [OR] = 10.2), renal disease (OR = 5.1), liver disease (OR = 4.8), metastatic cancer (OR = 4.6), pulmonary circulation

disorders (OR = 2.9), congestive heart failure (OR = 2.4), obesity
(OR = 2.1), non-metastatic malignancies (OR = 2.1), peripheral vascular
disorders (OR = 1.8), alcohol abuse (OR = 1.8), neurological disorders
(OR = 1.6), and cardiac arrhythmias (OR = 1.5). Increased length of
hospital stay among survivors was significantly predicted by paralysis
(90% increase), dementia (60%), peptic ulcer disease (53%), other neurological disorders (52%), HIV/AIDS (49%), renal disease (44%), a psychiatric diagnosis (42%), cerebrovascular disease (41%), cardiac arrhythmias
(40%), peripheral vascular disorders (39%), alcohol abuse (36%),
valvular disease (32%), liver disease (30%), diabetes (26%), congestive
heart failure (23%), drug abuse (20%), and hypertension (17%).

*Conclusions.*—A number of preexisting medical conditions influence
outcomes in acute burn injury. Patients with preburn HIV/AIDS, metastatic cancer, liver disease, and renal disease have particularly poor prognoses.

▶ The value of this study results from the fact that information on 31 338 adults
admitted to 70 burn centers in the American Burn Association were reviewed.
Given the large number of patients and the data, the information gleamed is
worthwhile. Not surprisingly, patients with comorbidities such as human immunodeficiency virus (HIV), renal disease, metastatic carcinoma, and liver disease,
had a particularly poor prognosis. It was surprising that the patients with
chronic pulmonary problems did not experience longer hospital stays or have
a negative change in mortality. For the practicing clinician it is important to
seek consultation early rather than late for patients who are admitted with
these particular problems to "beat the odds."

**R. E. Salisbury, MD**

**The Effect of Oxandrolone on the Endocrinologic, Inflammatory, and
Hypermetabolic Responses During the Acute Phase Postburn**
Jeschke MG, Finnerty CC, Suman OE, et al (Shriners Hosp for Children,
Galveston, TX)
*Ann Surg* 246:351-362, 2007

*Objective and Summary Background Data.*—Postburn long-term oxandrolone treatment improves hypermetabolism and body composition. The
effects of oxandrolone on clinical outcome, body composition, endocrine
system, and inflammation during the acute phase postburn in a large
prospective randomized single-center trial have not been studied.

*Methods.*—Burned children (n = 235) with >40% total body surface
area burn were randomized (block randomization 4:1) to receive standard
burn care (control, n = 190) or standard burn care plus oxandrolone for at
least 7 days (oxandrolone 0.1 mg/kg body weight q.12 hours p.o, n = 45).
Clinical parameters, body composition, serum hormones, and cytokine
expression profiles were measured throughout acute hospitalization.

Statistical analysis was performed by Student *t* test, or ANOVA followed by Bonferroni correction with significance accepted at *P* < 0.05.

*Results.*—Demographics and clinical data were similar in both groups. Length of intensive care unit stay was significantly decreased in oxandrolone-treated patients (0.48 ± 0.02 days/% burn) compared with controls (0.56 ± 0.02 days/% burn), (*P* < 0.05). Control patients lost 8 ± 1% of their lean body mass (LBM), whereas oxandrolone-treated patients had preserved LBM (+9 ± 4%), *P* < 0.05. Oxandrolone significantly increased serum prealbumin, total protein, testosterone, and AST/ALT, whereas it significantly decreased α2-macroglobulin and complement C3, *P* < 0.05. Oxandrolone did not adversely affect the endocrine and inflammatory response as we found no significant differences in the hormone panels and cytokine expression profiles.

*Conclusions.*—In this large prospective, double-blinded, randomized single-center study, oxandrolone shortened length of acute hospital stay, maintained LBM, improved body composition and hepatic protein synthesis while having no adverse effects on the endocrine axis postburn, but was associated with an increase in AST and ALT.

▶ This excellent article is a continuation of the work on metabolism in burn injury by the group at the Galveston Shriners Hospital. The efficacy of oxandrolone had been noted in adults in studies from Massachusetts General Hospital and this article shows its efficacy in children. For the sake of completeness, one should compare the positive and negative aspects of oxandrolone as opposed to human growth hormone.

**R. E. Salisbury, MD**

## Comparative evaluation of surface swab and quantitative full thickness wound biopsy culture in burn patients
Uppal SK, Ram S, Kwatra B, et al (Dayanand Med College & Hosp, Ludhiana, India; CMC & H, Ludhiana, India)
*Burns* 33:460-463, 2007

A total of 100 cases of burn were examined and screened bacteriologically for evidence of infection by surface swab culture, quantitative full thickness punch biopsy culture and blood culture. Gram negative organisms predominates the gram positive ones. Surface swab was found to correlate well with the biopsy as far the identification of causative organism is concerned. However, the latter technique was found to be more valuable as it also gives the critical load (>$10^5$CFU/g of tissue) of the organism beyond which metastatic invasion of the organism takes place (*p* < 0.01), thus obviating the repeated need for blood culture in burn patients.

▶ This article is a rehash of information gleamed almost 40 years ago by burn researchers. The bibliography in this article is highly inadequate and does not reflect extensive studies done by Heggers, Robson, and others. The value of the article is in making the newer generation of trainees aware of this work, which has great application, not just in burn patients but in all patients with wounds.

**R. E. Salisbury, MD**

---

### Vasopressin for the septic burn patient

Cartotto R, McGibney K, Smith T, et al (Ross Tilley Burn Centre, Toronto)
*Burns* 33:441-451, 2007

---

*Background.*—Exogenous arginine vasopressin (VP) has been increasingly used in the hemodynamic management of critically ill patients with septic shock, but its use in septic burn patients has not been systematically examined.

*Purpose.*—To review our experience with the use of VP in septic burn patients.

*Methods.*—Retrospective review of all patients who received VP at a tertiary care adult regional burn centre. Only patients who strictly met the American College of Chest Physicians/Society of Critical Care Medicine Consensus Criteria for sepsis at the time of VP initiation were analysed.

*Results.*—There were 30 septic burn patients treated on 43 distinct occasions with VP. This group had a mean (±S.D.) age of 49 ± 19 years, a mean % TBSA burn of 41 ± 15% and a 37% incidence of inhalation injury. A significant increase in mean arterial pressure (MAP), a significant decrease in heart rate (HR), and a trend towards increased urine output (UO) occurred following initiation of VP. When VP was added to an existing infusion of norepinephrine (NE), there was a significant NE sparing effect. VP was implicated in the death of one patient who developed diffuse upper gastrointestinal necrosis while on VP. Other complications in patients treated with VP included peripheral ischemia (2), skin graft failure (1) and donor site conversion (1). In all complications, VP had been administered in combination with prolonged NE infusions (mean of 10 µg/min over a mean of 177 h).

*Conclusion.*—VP is a useful adjunctive pressor that spares NE requirements in septic burn patients, but its use is not without risks, particularly when VP is combined with sustained moderate to high infusions of NE.

▶ This article is worth reading for multiple reasons. First, the discussion of the physiology of vasopressin (VP) and septic shock is worthwhile, as is the bibliography. The authors clearly state the unusual nature of this article in that VP was administered as the initial pressor agent. The result and complications make it obvious that this drug is not a first-line defender in the treatment of septic shock, and certainly should not be used by itself. In the burn patient with septic shock, the complications are formidable with loss of skin graft and donor site conversion.

**R. E. Salisbury, MD**

---

**Supraclavicular bilobed fasciocutaneous flap for postburn cervical contractures**
Ortiz CL, Carrasco AV, Torres AN, et al (Hosp Gen Universitario de Alicante, Spain)
*Burns* 33:770-775, 2007

---

Anterior cervical contractures after burn are a common problem in the treatment of sequelae in burnt patients. The contracture itself and the hypertrophic scarring can cause functional limitation and aesthetic disfigurement. As a consequence, the reconstruction of this area is a challenge to surgeons that must choose a procedure, which improves functionality and aesthetic appearance in addition to reversing the contracture, the surgical goal of avoiding a new scar band over time is added.

We present three patients with moderate (grade II) cervical contractures caused by suicide attempt and reconstructed by means of a bilobed flap based on the supraclavicular axis with the purpose of avoiding grafts in the donor area and performing it in a single procedure.

This flap is useful and reliable for reconstruction of defects caused by cervical scars in non-collaborative and psychologically unstable patients. The anatomy, surgical procedure and results in our series are presented in this article.

▶ This study nicely discusses the anterior cervical region contractures secondary to burn scars and the multiple possibilities for reconstruction. The key point is that the author identifies the type of case that is amenable to local flaps as opposed to release in skin graft or even a free flap reconstruction. His results appear very natural because he is using adjacent unburned skin of the same color and quality. Free flaps tend to look very bulky and unnatural and should be saved for salvage cases.

**R. E. Salisbury, MD**

---

**Flap choices to treat complex severe postburn hand contracture**
Ulkür E, Uygur F, Karagöz H, et al (Gulhane Military Med Academy, Istanbul, Turkey)
*Ann Plast Surg* 58:479-483, 2007

---

Many regions of the hand are affected seriously in the patients with complex severe postburn hand contractures. Multiple flap choices should be in count to treat complex severe postburn hand contractures affectively.

We preferred dorsal ulnar flap for palmar region, cross-finger flap, side finger flap, and combined use of both for flexion contracture of the fingers, and rhomboid flap for web contractures. Eight patients having complex severe postburn hand contractures were treated between November 2001 and February 2005. The maximum improvements of the joint extensions were 75 degrees for median of digits metacarpophalangeal joint and 105 degrees for proximal interphalangeal joint. Grasp function of the hand dramatically improved, and the bulk of the flap did not interfere grasping. Complex severe postburn hand contracture can be treated sufficiently with dorsal ulnar flap, combined use of cross-finger and side finger transposition flap, and rhomboid flap.

▶ This article describes several different flaps that have been successful in the hands of the surgeons for a total of 8 patients over a period of 5 years. This article is being reviewed because it elucidates multiple teaching points that young residents and attendings often overlook. First, flaps should not be the first alternative in correcting postburn hand contractures. Release of the contracture and split thickness skin grafting is a time-honored technique, which combined with nonsurgical modalities such as a compression glove, silicone and judicious splinting, yield superb results. Flaps are extremely important when, to achieve a release, one uncovers vital structures such as nerves, tendons, and joint surfaces. Secondly, the authors give no indication for why a particular operation was chosen or, indeed, why a flap was selected over skin grafting. Lastly, the authors talk about radically excising the contracture and scar tissue as being accepted treatment. The fact is that scar will remodel once a release is affected and it is not necessary to excise all the scar. Once the contracture is released and wound healing is achieved, the use of silicone and pressure dressings will result in softening of the surrounding skin, and especially the scar. Busy burn units that admit over 200 patients per year are regularly confronted with these types of problems, and it is worthwhile to have an algorithm of treatment that ranges from the simplest to the most complex with clear indications for why a surgical alternative is chosen.

**R. E. Salisbury, MD**

---

**Current concepts of microvascular reconstruction for limb salvage in electrical burn injuries**
Ofer N, Baumeister S, Megerle K, et al (Univ of Heidelberg, Germany)
*J Plast Reconstr Aesthetic Surg* 60:724-730, 2007

---

*Background.*—Microvascular reconstruction is rarely indicated in burn injuries. As the versatility and variability of free flaps have increased significantly during recent years so, the indications for this procedure have been expanded for limb salvage after electrical injuries.

*Methods.*—We report retrospectively the results of 26 free flaps for extremity reconstruction in 19 patients suffering from severe electrical burn injuries. Nine different free flap types were used. On the basis of this experience we were able to establish reconstructive principles in electrical injuries pertinent to the timing of reconstruction procedures.

*Results.*—Early coverage with muscular flaps was the most frequently used type of reconstruction. At a later stage of the treatment course reconstruction with cutaneous or fascial flaps was the preferred method; for the reconstruction of complex or multistructural defects ($n = 3$) combined 'chimeric' flaps were used.

Overall, the flap failure rate was 15% ($n = 4$). Interestingly, there was a relationship between flap failure rate and timing of the procedure. All the flap failures occurred within 5–21 days after trauma. No flap failure occurred during secondary reconstruction.

*Conclusions.*—Our data demonstrate that electrical burn injuries are distinct entities requiring individual reconstructive solutions for limb salvage. Even if our flap failure rate is relatively high it should not be forgotten that this type of reconstruction represents an opportunity for limb salvage as opposed to early amputation.

▶ This review article, 26 free flaps for extremity reconstruction, does not offer any new material, but is worth reviewing for several reasons. First, most reconstructive surgeons do not see high voltage electrical injuries requiring microvascular reconstruction, and this is a large series. The authors' experience is valuable, especially their high flap failure rate in early coverage situations. The bibliography provides an excellent review for those interested in the topic.

**R. E. Salisbury, MD**

---

## Increasing tendency in caustic esophageal burns and long-term polytetraflourethylene stenting in severe cases: 10 years experience

Atabek C, Surer I, Demirbag S, et al (Gulhane Military Med Academy, Ankara, Turkey)
*J Pediatr Surg* 42:636-640, 2007

---

In recent years, lye products have come into common household use in Turkey. Unfortunately, we have noted more cases of serious corrosive esophagitis owing to accidental caustic agent ingestion. The aims of this study were to (1) evaluate our experience with these cases and (2) investigate the effects of long-term intraesophageal polytetrafluorethylene stenting on esophageal remodeling and its impact upon the need for esophageal replacement. Between 1997 and 2006, 68 patients (44 males and 22 females) with accidental caustic agent ingestion were admitted to our department, the only tertiary care referral center for the Turkish Army. Once stabilized, esophagoscopy was performed for injury grading (grades 0, 1, 2a, 3b, 3a, or 3b) as described by Millar and Cywes (*Pediatric Surgery.* 1998;969-979). Esophagogram was performed 3 weeks after injury to assess healing. At presentation, the injury grade for 24, 31, 11, and 1 cases were 0 or 1, 2a, 2b, and 3a, respectively. One case had gastric outlet obstruction. All cases of grade 0 or 1 injuries had a normal esophagogram at 3 weeks postinjury. For the remaining 44 patients, several treatment modalities have been applied, including antegrade and retrograde dilatations in 31 grade 2a patients, intraluminal stenting in 11 grade 2b patients, esophageal reconstruction in 1 grade 3a patient, and gastroenterostomy in 1. Of the 11 patients with esophageal stenting, 8 patients have resumed a normal diet after 9 to 14 months of stenting. Mean follow up duration is 3.5 years (1-6 years) after stent removal. In the remaining 3 cases, treatment is still ongoing. Esophagitis and esophageal structuring because of caustic agent ingestion is a major public health problem in Turkey. Our small uncontrolled pilot series suggests that intraluminal polytetrafluorethylene stenting may be an effective treatment method to reduce the need for major surgical reconstruction of recalcitrant esophageal strictures.

▶ This series from Turkey involves 68 patients over 9 years. Eleven patients required esophageal stenting and 8 of these resumed a normal diet after 9 to 14 months. The authors believe that their intraluminal polytetraflourethylene stent might well be an effective treatment in reducing the need for major surgical reconstruction for someone with persistent esophageal stricture. Considering the morbidity of this problem, their results are excellent, as is the bibliography. This condition is not common and reviewing their classification and their indications for surgical intervention may be very worthwhile for the practitioner seeing his first case.

**R. E. Salisbury, MD**

---

**The Scalp Is an Advantageous Donor Site for Thin-Skin Grafts: A Report on 945 Harvested Samples**
Mimoun M, Chaouat M, Picovski D, et al (Rothschild Hosp, Paris; Saint-Antoine Hosp, Paris)
*Plast Reconstr Surg* 118:369-373, 2006

---

*Background.*—Thin-skin grafts taken from the thigh or buttock take a long time to heal and leave permanent scars.

*Methods.*—The authors conducted a retrospective study based on their experience with 945 thin-skin grafts (0.2 mm) taken from the scalps of 757 adult patients between January of 1999 and December of 2003.

*Results.*—Of the 757 patients, 89 had grafts taken repeatedly from the scalp. The mean healing time was 6.2 days for a single harvest and 10.2 days for repeated (same hospitalization) harvests. During follow-up, eight patients had microalopecia and three developed "concrete scalp deformity." Of these 11 patients, eight had undergone repeated harvests. None of the other patients had any scarring; they were completely healed by day 15.

*Conclusions.*—The results of this study confirm the rapidity of scalp healing compared with other donor sites. Providing patients with clear, detailed explanations helps minimize the psychological impact of having their heads shaved, and a rigorous technique can contain the two major potential risks: hemorrhage and alopecia. The adult scalp seems to be a donor site to be exploited whenever possible.

▶ This article summarizes the authors' extensive experience using the scalp skin graft donor site. They remind us all that this is a valuable skin graft donor site. I agree that it provides good skin and heals with a hidden scar. However, it is not without problems. Most patients hate to have their head shaved. The prolonged time period of re-epithelialization coupled with hair growth into the healing wound makes this a donor site that usually heals more slowly than average. Although I have many colleagues who love this donor site, I seldom use it.

**W. L. Garner, MD**

## A retrospective cohort study of Acticoat™ versus Silvazine™ in a paediatric population

Cuttle L, Naidu S, Mill J, et al (Univ of Queensland, Herston, Australia)
*Burns* 33:701-707, 2007

We wished to determine whether changing our centre's practice of using Acticoat™ instead of Silvazine™ as our first-line burns dressing provided a better standard of care in terms of efficacy, cost and ease of use. A retrospective cohort study was performed examining 328 Silvazine™ treated patients from January 2000 to June 2001 and 241 Acticoat™ treated patients from July 2002 to July 2003. During those periods the respective dressings were used exclusively. There was no significant difference in age, %BSA and mechanism of burn between the groups. In the Silvazine™ group, 25.6% of children required grafting compared to 15.4% in the Acticoat™ group ($p = 0.001$). When patients requiring grafting were excluded, the time taken for re-epithelialisation in the Acticoat™ group (14.9 days) was significantly less than that for the Silvazine™ group (18.3 days), $p = 0.047$. There were more wounds requiring long term scar management in the Silvazine™ group (32.6%) compared to the Acticoat™ group (29.5%), however this was not significant. There was only one positive blood culture in each group, indicating that both Silvazine™ and Acticoat™ are potent antimicrobial agents. The use of Acticoat™ as our primary burns dressing has dramatically changed our clinical practice. Inpatients are now only 18% of the total admissions, with the vast majority of patients treated on an outpatient basis. In terms of cost, Acticoat™ was demonstrated to be less expensive over the treatment period than Silvazine™. We have concluded that Acticoat™ is a safe, cost-effective, efficacious dressing that reduces the time for re-epithelialisation and the requirement for grafting and long term scar management, compared to Silvazine™.

▶ Although this is a retrospective study, there are several interesting results that are worth noting. First, there is no increased incidence of positive blood cultures in the Acticoat™ group. Secondly, costs were contained and, in fact, improved by the use of the Acticoat™ in converting many patients to outpatient status. Unquestionably, the dressing with Acticoat™ is less painful for the children than using Silvazene™, and doing more frequent dressing changes. What is most surprising and difficult to understand is why the Acticoat™-treated group seemed to heal more rapidly? Perhaps this aspect of the study warrants further investigation.

**R. E. Salisbury, MD**

---

**Acticoat Versus Allevyn as a Split-Thickness Skin Graft Donor-Site Dressing: A Prospective Comparative Study**
Argirova M, Hadjiski O, Victorova A (Emergency Med Inst "Pirogov," Sofia, Bulgaria)
*Ann Plast Surg* 59:415-422, 2007

---

The study comprises 27 operated patients with similar burns. Fifteen donor sites treated with Acticoat (Smith & Nephew) and 12 donor sites treated with Allevyn (Smith & Nephew) have been analyzed with respect to epithelization time, antibacterial effect, ease of dressing change, pain, and pharmacologic and cost-effective characteristics. All donor sites after the reepithelization were evaluated using the Vancouver Scar Scale for the assessment of scars at the fourth, eighth, and 12th weeks. The obtained results demonstrate statistically significant faster epithelization ($P = 0.012$ on the eighth day and $P = 0.0081$ on the 10th day) and better comfort for the patient with the Acticoat dressing ($P < 0.05$). With regard to bacterial growth ($P > 0.05$) there is no statistically significant difference in the application of Acticoat and Allevyn. The Vancouver Scar Scale assessment shows no statistically significant difference ($P > 0.05$) in the application of both Acticoat and Allevyn. There is no considerable difference in the cost of treatment between both dressings. The results obtained determine both dressings as suitable for application on donor sites. If there is a possibility of choice, the Acticoat dressing is preferable.

▶ We have too few comparative trials in Plastic Surgery, so these authors should be congratulated on a study of one of our very common problems. This is important because donor site dressings are a source of profound argument, bias, and conjecture, all with little useful comparative information. The answer? Simply that an antimicrobial dressing works better than an absorbent dressing. Why would this be so? There's increasing information that low levels of bacteria contribute to inflammation within the wound and that this inflammation inhibits wound healing. The use of a topical antimicrobial can significantly prevent this. Dressing a wound with an antibiotic piece of an adherent gauze is a partial solution but the ability to release silver, as the Acticoat material does for the duration of wound healing, has significant, theoretical and practical benefits. In this case, those benefits are proven in patients. I'm happy to tell anyone who will listen that we treat all of our donor sites with a silver releasing dressing and pick between the ones currently available based on cost and particular characteristic which we are seeking: adherence, desire to re-evaluate the wound, and current pricing within our university health care system. All seem to do better than our previous donor site dressings, and I hope you will consider trying them. Yes, they cost more than a dry piece of Xeroform, but then they work better.

**W. L. Garner, MD**

---

**Reducing susceptibility to bacteremia after experimental burn injury: a role for selective decontamination of the digestive tract**
Horton JW, Maass DL, White J, et al (Univ of Texas Southwestern Med Ctr, Dallas)
*J Appl Physiol* 102:2207-2216, 2007

---

We proposed that selective decontamination of the digestive tract (SDD) initiated after experimental burn injury would decrease myocardial inflammation and dysfunction after a second insult such as septic challenge. Rats were divided into eight experimental groups. Groups included sham burn plus sham sepsis, burn alone, sepsis alone, and burn plus sepsis given either water by oral gavage for 5 days after burn (or sham burn) or given oral antibiotics (polymyxin E, 15 mg; tobramycin, 6 mg; 5-flucytosin, 100 mg given by oral gavage, 2× daily for 5 days after burn or sham burn). Cardiac function and inflammation were studied 24 h after septic challenge. In the absence of SDD, burn alone, sepsis alone, or burn plus septic challenge promoted cardiac myocyte secretion of TNF-α (burn, 174 ± 11; sepsis, 269 ± 19; burn + sepsis, 453 ± 14 pg/ml), IL-1β (burn, 35 ± 2; sepsis, 29 ± 1; burn + sepsis, 48 ± 7 pg/ml), and IL-6 (burn, 143 ± 18; sepsis, 116 ± 3; burn + sepsis, 248 ± 12 pg/ml) compared with values measured in sham (TNF-α, 3 ± 1; IL-1β, 1 ± 0.4; IL-6, 6 ± 1.5 pg/ml) ($P < 0.05$). Impaired ventricular contraction and relaxation responses were evident in the absence of SDD [burn + sepsis: left ventricular pressure (LVP), 65 ± 4 mmHg; rate of LVP rise (+dP/d$t$), 1,320 ± 131 mmHg/s compared with values measured in sham: LVP, 96 ± 4 mmHg; +dP/d$t$, 2,095 ± 99 mmHg/s, $P < 0.05$]. SDD treatment of experimental burn attenuated septic challenge-related inflammatory responses and improved myocardial contractile responses, producing cardiac TNF-α, IL-1β, and IL-6 levels, LVP, +dP/d$t$, and rate of LVP fall (−dP/d$t$) values that were significantly better ($P < 0.05$) than values measured in burn plus sepsis in the absence of SDD. This work confirms that endogenous gut organisms contribute to sensitivity to subsequent infectious challenge.

▶ This experimental rat model infection article is of interest because of the questions it raises rather than the answers that it provides. The authors indicate that selective gut decontamination with antibiotics increases the inflammatory response that occurs with a septic challenge. They rightly do not attempt to extrapulate their findings to the human condition. In fact, they mention that other studies showed that decontamination of the digestive tract gave rise to resistant organisms. The reviewers' greatest concern is the fact that there are no articles in the bibliography before 1983. There is a widespread tendency of younger investigators to forget that they are standing on the shoulders of others and that no meaningful studies were performed before the widespread use of the computer and computer searches. Multiple studies from a generation ago clearly elucidated that burns are a multisystem disease. The prophylactic use of antibiotics has always given rise to resistant organisms, resulting in sepsis, or the emergence of opportunistic invaders such as fungi, which take over an ecological niche vacated by the indiscriminant use of antibiotics. For those intellectually inclined to understand the profession, background reading worked on by their illustrious predecessors is a must.

R. E. Salisbury, MD

---

**Arteriovenous $CO_2$ Removal Improves Survival Compared to High Frequency Percussive and Low Tidal Volume Ventilation in a Smoke/Burn Sheep Acute Respiratory Distress Syndrome Model**
Schmalstieg FC, Keeney SE, Rudloff HE, et al (Univ of Texas Med Branch, Galveston)
*Ann Surg* 246:512-523, 2007

---

*Objectives and Summary Background.*—Low tidal volume ventilation (LTV) has improved survival with acute respiratory distress syndrome (ARDS) by reducing lung stretch associated with volutrauma and barotrauma. Additional strategies to reduce lung stretch include arteriovenous carbon dioxide removal ($AVCO_2R$), and high frequency percussive ventilation (HFPV). We performed a prospective, randomized study comparing these techniques in our clinically relevant $LD_{100}$ sheep model of ARDS to compare survival, pathology, and inflammation between the 3 ventilator methods.

*Methods.*—Adult sheep (n = 61) received smoke inhalation (48 breaths) and a 40% third-degree burn. After ARDS developed ($Pao_2/FiO_2$ <200), animals were randomized. In experiment 1, animals were killed at 48 hours after randomization. Hemodynamics, pulmonary function, injury scores, myeloperoxidase (MPO) in lung tissues and neutrophils, IL-8 in lung tissues, and apoptosis were evaluated. In experiment 2, the end point was survival to 72 hours after onset of ARDS or end-of-life criteria with extension of the same studies performed in experiment 1.

*Results.*—There were no differences in hemodynamics, but minute ventilation was lower in the $AVCO_2R$ group and Paco2 for the HFPV and $AVCO_2R$ animals remained lower than LTV. Airway obstruction and injury scores were not different among the 3 ventilation strategies. In experiment 1, lung tissue MPO and IL-8 were not different among the ventilation strategies. However, in experiment 2, lung tissue MPO was significantly lower for $AVCO_2R$-treated animals ($AVCO_2R < HFPV < LTV$). TUNEL staining showed little DNA breakage in neutrophils from experiment 1, but significantly increased breakage in all 3 ventilator strategies in experiment 2. In contrast, $AVCO_2R$ tissue neutrophils showed significant apoptosis at 72 hours post-ARDS criteria as measured by nuclear condensation ($P < 0.001$). Survival 72 hours post-ARDS criteria was highest for $AVCO_2R$ (71%) compared with HFPV (55%) and LTV (33%) ($AVCO_2R$ vs. LTV, $P = 0.05$).

*Conclusions.*—Significantly more animals survived $AVCO_2R$ than LTV. In experiment 2, Lung MPO was significantly lower for $AVCO_2R$, compared with LTV ($P < 0.05$). This finding taken together with the TUNEL and neutrophil apoptosis results, suggested that disposition of neutrophils 72 hours post-ARDS criteria was different among the ventilatory strategies with neutrophils from $AVCO_2R$-treated animals removed chiefly through apoptosis, but in the cases of HFPV and LTV, dying by necrosis in lung tissue.

▶ This article is extremely important, as is the bibliography, in attempting to understand pulmonary dynamics. There is so much experimental data in the literature done in models that have no relevance to humans. Significantly, this study was done on large animals and is clinically relevant. This article begs for clinical human follow-up.

**R. E. Salisbury, MD**

# 4 Hand and Upper Extremity

**The reverse posterior interosseous flap and its composite flap: Experience with 201 flaps**

Lu L-j, Gong X, Lu X-m, et al (Ji Lin Univ, Chang Chun, PR China; Third People's Hosp of Yang Quan City, Shan Xin)
*J Plast Reconstr Aesthetic Surg* 60:876-882, 2007

---

*Objective.*—To introduce our experiences of using the reverse posterior interosseous flap and its composite flap.

*Methods.*—In the series of 201 cases, the fasciocutaneous flap was used to cover skin defects over the distal 1/3rd forearm, wrist and hand in 174 cases. The composite flap with the vascularised ulna bone graft was used to reconstruct the thumbs in 11 cases, and with the vascularised tendon graft was used to repair tendon defects with skin defects in 16 cases. The size of the ulna graft was 3–6 cm in length and 1–2 cm in width. The 4–7 cm tendon graft was obtained from the extensor digiti quinti or extensor carpi ulnaris. The size of the flaps ranged from 5 cm × 4 cm to 16 cm × 10 cm.

*Results.*—One flap failed completely. Of the other 200 flaps which survived 16 cases had venous congestion and had partial necrosis at the distal end. The size of the necrotic area ranged from 1 to 4 cm in length. Ninety-three patients were followed up for at least 6 months, and included 10 patients with composite flaps. Generally, the flap matched the surrounding skin. But 10 cases had a lipectomy. The sensibility did not recover or achieved S1 within 6 months. For the extensor tendon defect, the function of finger extension was nearly normal and tenolysis was not required. In contrast, tenolysis was required after the flexor tendon reconstruction. However, these patients refused surgery. The bone grafts were healed in 3 months. The reconstructed thumb looked abnormal and lacked normal sensibility, although the patients used them. The linear scar line was conspicuous over the dorsum of the forearm.

*Conclusion.*—The reverse posterior interosseous flap is a reliable method to cover skin defects over the distal 1/3rd of the forearm, the wrist and hand. The composite flap with a vascularised tendon graft is an optimal reconstructive option for any extensor tendon loss (III zone) associated with a skin defect. Using the composite flap with a vascularised bone graft or combined with the digital neurovascular flap is another way to reconstruct the thumb.

▶ The authors present this extensive series of 201 posterior interosseous flaps. The article is clearly written and nicely analyzed. The results are excellent. What is missing is critical analysis of where this flap fits in the overall options for upper extremity surgery. We know that these authors are proficient with this flap. We do not know where they use other flaps in preference to this one. Outcomes and best practices are the next step.

**D. J. Smith, Jr, MD**

---

**Functional gracilis flap in thenar reconstruction**
Baker PA, Watson SB (Glasgow Royal Infirmary, Scotland)
*J Plast Reconstr Aesthetic Surg* 60:828-834, 2007

---

Restoration of lost opposition in the context of significant thenar soft tissue defects represents a tremendous reconstructive challenge. Free functioning muscle transfer has been described in this context and has the advantage of providing both a functioning muscle unit as well as soft tissue coverage in a single reconstructive procedure. It adds to the injured limb, and by sparing donor tendons avoids the need for re-education of motor function. We describe the use of a free innervated gracilis muscle flap for functional thenar reconstruction in two unique cases following extensive traumatic loss of thenar skin and musculature. Crucially, in each case, the recurrent motor branch of the median nerve had been destroyed at its point of insertion into the thenar muscle remnants.

*Aim.*—To date, the main reported disadvantages of free functioning muscle transfer in thenar reconstruction include difficult flap dissections, donor site morbidity, inadequate strength and excursion of the transplanted muscle and excessively bulky flaps. Our aim was, as far as possible, to address these issues.

*Surgical Procedure.*—Each thenar defect was measured and a corresponding segment of gracilis muscle, measured in situ, was raised on the proximal neurovascular pedicle. End-side microvascular anastomosis was performed between the medial circumflex femoral artery and the radial artery. The venae comitantes of the pedicle were anastomosed end-end with those of the radial artery and also with the cephalic vein. Epineural anastomosis was performed between the motor branch of the obturator nerve and the recurrent motor branch of the median nerve. Each flap was covered with a split thickness skin graft.

*Results.*—Both flaps survived without any complication. Both patients regained excellent voluntary thumb opposition, sufficient to allow return to full-time employment, and had restoration of sufficient thenar bulk. This was achieved with minimal donor site morbidity.

*Conclusions.*—Restoration of lost opposition, in the context of significant thenar soft tissue defects, can be achieved using a free functional gracilis flap. This produces clinically excellent functional results and can be carried out as a single stage reconstructive procedure. This is a novel application of a tremendously versatile donor muscle in functioning free muscle transfer.

▶ Most abstracts I pick try to support large series and long-term follow-ups. This abstract is a notable exception. Only 2 cases, but what an eloquent solution to a difficult problem. Most of us would probably embark on local/regional multistage solutions. These authors forsake the "reconstructive ladder" and go directly to the top. They end up with a unique, single stage solution that is for many reasons superior to "traditional" procedures. This is a superior application for a functional free muscle transfer.

**D. J. Smith, Jr, MD**

## Current Practice of Microsurgery by Members of the American Society for Surgery of the Hand

Payatakes AH, Zagoreos NP, Fedorcik GG, et al (Duke Univ, Durham, NC)
*J Hand Surg* 32:541-547, 2007

*Purpose.*—First, to determine the percentage of members of the American Society for Surgery of the Hand (ASSH) that use microsurgical techniques as part of their surgery practice, and second, to identify factors limiting their use of these techniques.

*Methods.*—A 34-item, anonymous, Web-based survey was sent to all active ASSH members. Twelve items concerned demographics and 22 items addressed prior microsurgical training, current use of these techniques, factors currently limiting their use of these techniques, and potential methods to address these limiting factors.

*Results.*—Responses were received from 561 of 1,238 of the ASSH members contacted (45% response rate). Most had residency training in orthopedics (N = 460, 82%) or plastic surgery (N = 79, 14%), followed by a hand fellowship in an orthopedic (N = 363, 62%) or combined program (N = 170, 30%). More than 54% (N = 304) practiced privately, 33% (N = 184) practiced in tertiary institutions, and the remainder practiced at regional centers. Of those responding, 505 (90%) stated that hand surgery constituted more than 50% of their practice, whereas for 527 (94%) respondents microsurgery comprised less than 25%. Most members (N = 398, 71%) accepted emergency patients, of which 223 (56%) at a referral center. Three hundred sixteen respondents (56%) performed replantations, of whom 196 (62%) performed fewer than 5 per year. Four hundred fifteen respondents (74%) observed a decrease in replantation attempts over the past decade. This was attributed to refinement of indications (N = 17, 83%), fewer patients with amputations (N = 116, 28%), and declining reimbursement (N = 344, 4%). Reasons for not personally performing replantations included busy elective schedules (N = 125, 51%), inadequate confidence in performing replantations (N = 96, 39%), and disappointment in results (N = 56, 23%). Thirty percent (N = 74) stated they would reconsider performing replantations if reimbursement was greater. Practice rates of examined microsurgical procedures ranged from 22% to 57%, although most had received microsurgical training. Despite rating their fellowship as excellent (N = 393, 70%) or good (N = 135, 24%), only 315 (56%) considered their present microsurgical skills to be above average. Many respondents believed that they would benefit from continuous training through continuing education courses.

*Conclusions.*—Educational, economic, and practical factors discourage the clinical application of microsurgical technique by hand surgeons. This unfavorable environment should be addressed by policy-making organizations and continuous surgical training.

*Type of Study/Level of Evidence.*—Other/Survey.

▶ The authors try to assess replantation surgery as a barometer for microsurgery. I believe they may have drawn the wrong conclusion. The focus, as is nicely outlined in the article, is on replantation, reimbursement, and call. Microsurgery is passively evaluated as the sine qua non. What we don't know is how many of those not doing replants may be doing elective microsurgery. With the advent of perforator flaps, more centers are reporting large series of free tissue transfers. The data is troubling if many of us are limiting our practice and avoiding microsurgery. But as presented, I believe this is a condemnation of call, call pay, and reimbursement, not microsurgical incorporation into our practice.

**D. J. Smith, Jr, MD**

---

### A Retrospective Analysis of 154 Arterialized Venous Flaps for Hand Reconstruction: An 11-Year Experience
Woo S-H, Kim K-C, Lee G-J, et al (Yeungnam Univ, Daegu, Korea)
*Plast Reconstr Surg* 119:1823-1838, 2007

---

*Background.*—The purpose of this study was to present the authors' 11-year clinical experience involving 154 cases of arterialized venous flaps for hand reconstruction.

*Methods.*—The authors classified the venous flaps based on their size and composition. According to their size, flaps smaller than 10 cm² were classified as small (*n* = 48), flaps larger than 25 cm² were classified as large (*n* = 42), and those in between were classified as medium (*n* = 64). Classified according to their composition, there were 88 cases (57.1

percent) of venous skin flaps, 28 cases (18.2 percent) of innervated venous flaps, 15 cases (9.7 percent) of tendocutaneous venous flaps, and 17 cases (11 percent) of conduit venous flaps to repair arterial defects. There were six cases (3.9 percent) of composite venous flaps.

*Results.*—The success rate of the flap transfer was 98.1 percent. The incidence of partial flap necrosis was 5.2 percent. The mean number of included veins was 2.17 for a small flap, 2.60 for a medium-sized flap, and 4.07 for a large flap ($p < 0.01$). The mean area of flap necrosis was 45.0 percent, 31.67 percent, and 18.75 percent for small, medium, and large flaps, respectively ($p = 0.807$). In eight cases of innervated venous flaps, the average static two-point discrimination was 10 mm (range, 8 to 15 mm). In 12 cases of tendocutaneous venous flaps, active range of motion at the proximal interphalangeal, distal interphalangeal, and metacarpophalangeal joints was 60, 20, and 75 degrees, respectively.

*Conclusions.*—The authors conclude that the arterialized venous flap is a valuable and effective tool for reconstructing complex hand injuries and may have a more comprehensive set of indications.

▶ One hundred fifty-four flaps, 11 years experience, 98.1% success rate—sounds like something I should adopt and clearly champion in resident teaching. But I don't! The arterialized venous flap has not been endorsed by most in the plastic surgical community. The ability to provide large thin flaps is appealing. The results are impressive, but I think most of us are confused by the physiology. The author acknowledges significant edema, swelling, and blistering in the first week. For those of us not familiar with the flap, this equates to flap failure. Why would we purposefully do this? Perforator flaps make more physiologic and anatomic sense even if they may require a second operation.

**D. J. Smith, Jr, MD**

---

**The use of integra artificial dermis to minimize donor-site morbidity after suprafascial dissection of the radial forearm flap**
Gravvanis AI, Tsoutsos DA, Iconomou T, et al (Gen State Hosp of Athens, Greece)
*Microsurgery* 27:583-587, 2007

---

In an effort to minimize the radial forearm flap donor-site morbidity, the flap was elevated using the suprafascial dissection technique, in six patients with various facial defects. The donor site was covered primarily with Integra artificial skin and secondarily with an ultrathin split-thickness skin graft. The mean time to wound healing of the forearm donor site was 24 days. There were no flap failures, and all flaps healed uneventfully. At the end of the follow-up, all patients showed normal range of motion of the wrist and the fingers, normal power grip, and power pinch. All patients evaluated the esthetic appearance of the forearm donor site as very good. In conclusion, suprafascial dissection of the forearm flap creates a superior graft recipient site, and the use of Integra artificial dermis is a valuable advancement to further minimize the donor-site morbidity, resulting in excellent functional and aesthetic outcomes.

▶ I love Integra for its benefits in my acute and reconstructive burn practice and want to disclose that I am on their speaker's panel. In this context, this use of Integra is a clever idea to decrease the morbidity of radial forearm flap donor sites. It helps the contour irregularity. It allows closure and coverage of the flexor carpi radialis tendon if it becomes exposed. The disadvantage is, of course, a 2-stage reconstruction. Given the hassle of a second procedure a month later, I think you will be happy with how well this product can solve this donor site difficulty.

**W. L. Garner, MD**

# 5  Aesthetic

## Eyelids

### Peribulbar Anesthesia for Blepharoplasty

Lessa S, Passarelli CA (Univ of Rio de Janeiro, Brazil; Pró-Oftalmo, Rio de Janeiro, Brazil)
*Aesthetic Plast Surg* 31:463-466, 2007

*Background.*—Peribulbar anesthesia for inferior blepharoplasty was used successfully in 788 selected cases over the past 9 years. This technique is largely accepted for ophthalmologic procedures, but is not yet specifically used for blepharoplasty.

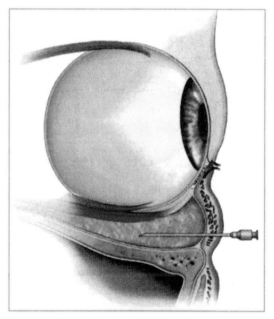

FIGURE 6.—Lateral view. The needle is positioned a depth of 31 mm, just beyond the globe equator, thereby preventing optic nerve and muscular cone trauma. (Reprinted from Lessa S, Passarelli CA. Peribulbar anesthesia for blepharoplasty. *Aesthetic Plast Surg.* 2007;31:463-466, with permission from the Springer Science+Business Media LLC.)

*Methods.*—In the past 9 years, 788 patients ages 36 to 77 years were submitted to inferior peribulbar anesthesia for blepharoplasty procedures. Of these patients, 623 (79%) were women and 165 (21%) were men. The anesthetic procedure is performed using a needle introduced at the junction of the medial two-thirds and the lateral third of the inferior orbital rim (point A). With the patient staring forward, the needle is introduced through the lid at point A. It enters the orbital cavity just above the orbital floor periosteum until the globe equator is minimally trespassed (depth, ~31 mm). There, 3 ml of the local anesthetic solution (2% lidocaine + 0.5% bupivacaine) is slowly injected.

*Results.*—None of our treated patients reported pain or discomfort during or after the surgical procedure. Immediately after inferior peribulbar anesthesia, chemosis was observed in 17 cases (2.2%) and orbital hematoma in 3 cases (0.4%). Diplopia, or a slight imaging distortion lasting a few hours may occur after inferior peribulbar anesthesia.

*Conclusion.*—Inferior peribulbar anesthesia for blepharoplasty offers surprising results. The surgical procedures are performed pain free, leaving the patients completely relaxed and allowing an easier surgical procedure. This technique should be performed only by highly skilled anesthesiologists or surgeons with a perfect knowledge of the complex orbital anatomy (Figs 6 and 7).

▶ The distortion by direct injection of local anesthesia in blepharoplasty patients can be overcome by Whitease, which allows dispersion of the edema. It can also be overcome with experience, which allows for adjustments

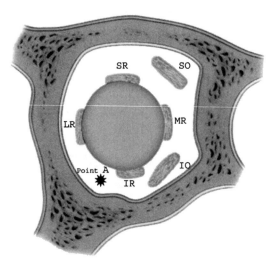

FIGURE 7.—Frontal view. Point A location avoids ocular extrinsic muscle insertions during needle introduction. (Reprinted from Lessa S, Passarelli CA. Peribulbar anesthesia for blepharoplasty. *Aesthetic Plast Surg*. 2007;31:463-466, with permission from the Springer Science+Business Media LLC.)

in the surgeon's eye to the distortion that results. The issue of pain with fat excision is a matter that this technique overcomes; however, a needle 31 mm into the socket is not a problem unless you do not know the anatomy. Also, one must realize that these deeper injections may give temporary strabismus, an alteration of the pupil, which can be alarming.

**P. W. McKinney, MD, CM**

---

**Eyelid phenol peel: An important adjunct to blepharoplasty**
Gatti JE (Univ of Med and Dentistry of New Jersey, Cherry Hill)
*Ann Plast Surg* 60:14-18, 2008

---

Deep peeling with phenol solutions has been criticized because of the hypopigmentation that usually results. The lower eyelid skin, after routine blepharoplasty, will retain its hyper-pigmentation and fine wrinkles. Phenol peeling of the lower eyelid will produce a complementary lightening of the skin and improvement in the wrinkling. This report explains the technique, used by the author, to improve blepharoplasty results.

▶ The author points out that eyelids can be peeled, but if a skin flap has been used for a blepharoplasty it must not be done at the time of the original operation because of the risk of full thickness skin loss. We published an article in 1991 entitled "The Fourth Option,"[1] and we did a phenol peel at the time of surgery, but only in those patients on whom we used a skin muscle flap. Phenol tightens eyelids skin and reduces wrinkles, but in the long run, it will lighten the skin. It can, like any other burn by any other method, whether it is heat, chemical, or sandpapering, make the skin crepe-like because a burn is a burn and some scar tissue is produced. Therefore, burning techniques should be used sparingly when you consider the long-range interests of the patient.

**P. W. McKinney, MD, CM**

*Reference*

1. McKinney P, Zukowki ML, Mossie R. The fourth option: a novel approach to lower lid blepharoplasty. *Aesthetic Plast Surg.* 1991;15:293-296.

---

**Power of the Pinch: Pinch Lower Lid Blepharoplasty**
Kim EM, Bucky LP (Univ of Pennsylvania, Philadelphia)
*Ann Plast Surg* 60:532-537, 2008

---

Lower lid blepharoplasty is performed with great variation in technique. Conventional lower lid blepharoplasty with anterior fat removal, via the orbital septum, has a potential lower lid malposition rate of 15% to 20%. Lower lid malposition and the stigma of obvious lower lid surgery have led plastic surgeons to continue to change their approach to lower lid rejuvenation. In recent years, some surgeons have come to rely on alternative procedures like laser resurfacing alone or in conjunction with transconjunctival fat removal and canthopexy in an effort to avoid such complications. The pinch blepharoplasty technique removes redundant skin without undermining. This allows for more controlled wound healing, predictable recovery, and potential for simultaneous laser resurfacing. The combination of pinch blepharoplasty with transconjunctival fat removal leaves the middle lamella intact and reduces the chance of scleral show or ectropion. The purpose of this series is to demonstrate that pinch excision of redundant lower eyelid skin can be safely performed, and that it can be used with laser resurfacing and/or transconjunctival fat removal for optimal treatment of the aging eye. A retrospective review of 46 consecutive patients who underwent pinch blepharoplasty, either in isolation or with other periorbital procedures, was performed. Follow-up was at least 4 months (range of 4–24 months). In addition, we performed a prospective study of 25 consecutive patients to quantify the amount of skin removed and evaluate results and complications. An average of 8 mm of skin was resected (range of 4–12 mm) with the pinch blepharoplasty technique. Of these patients, 5.6% also underwent transconjunctival blepharoplasty, laser resurfacing, and/or fat grafting of the nasojugal groove. Despite the addition of simultaneous laser resurfacing, we did not see an increase in lower lid malposition. Three of the 71 patients had temporary scleral show that resolved with lower lid massage. In total, only 4 patients had isolated pinch lower lid blepharoplasty. Twelve patients had orbicularis suspension and 15 had either canthopexy or canthoplasty. Five patients who had orbicularis suspension, canthopexy, or canthoplasty had periorbital edema. Two also had pronounced chemosis. Four patients had mild rounding of the lower lid. Pinch blepharoplasty is a versatile technique that produces consistent results. This study confirms that more skin from the lower lid can be resected than classically described. Pinch blepharoplasty can be performed safely in combination with other procedures to enhance lower lid appearance. The absence of skin undermining allows for safe simultaneous laser resurfacing. Preserving the middle lamella and supporting it when necessary, allows one to resect significant amounts of lower lid skin without significant risk of scleral show, lower lid rounding, and ectropion. Patients with poor lid tone or laxity may benefit from supportive procedures such as the canthopexy or canthoplasty.

▶ Over 300 patients, over an 8-year period, studied a procedure that evolved from reconstructive work in Graves's disease. Techniques to tighten the lower lid have relied on oblique vectors placing the tension in the region of the lateral canthus either by ligament, tarsal plate tightening, or mid face suspensions. Application of vertical tension was limited because tension on the lid margin may cause, at the least, sclera show. Using Lockwood's ligaments (see Fig 1 and Fig 3 in the original article) as a suspensory support for vertical tension, did not lead to ectropion or scleral show in this series. The patients illustrated were all in their 40s. Would similar results be obtained with fat sparing operations without Lockwood's suspension? To me, the use in older patients would demonstrate the potential of this technique, which begins to show its suspension strength with its tear trough correction (see Fig 10 in the original article). It is not clear if only suspension with fat sparing was used, or if fat was placed in the trough. This is an intriguing technique with a vertical vector for suspension of the lower lid.

**P. W. McKinney, MD, CM**

### Treatment of Lower Eyelid Malposition with Dermis Fat Grafting

Korn BS, Kikkawa DO, Cohen SR, et al (Shiley Eye Ctr Univ of California, San Diego; Univ of California, San Diego; et al)
*Ophthalmology* 115:744.e2-751.e2, 2008

*Purpose.*—To report a new technique in the repair of lower eyelid malposition using dermis fat as a posterior lamellar spacer graft.

*Design.*—Retrospective, consecutive, nonrandomized interventional case series.

*Participants.*—Eleven patients who underwent surgical correction for symptomatic lower eyelid malposition using dermis fat as a spacer graft.

*Methods.*—Patients with symptomatic lower eyelid malposition after blepharoplasty, trauma, craniofacial syndromes, and human immunodeficiency virus-associated lipodystrophy were treated with midfacial lifting, combined with dermis fat posterior lamellar spacer grafting.

*Main Outcome Measures.*—Preoperative and postoperative measurements of eyelid position, margin-to-reflex distance (defined as the distance from the upper eyelid to the central corneal light reflex, and the distance from the lower eyelid to the corneal light reflex), lagophthalmos, corneal staining, presence of ocular surface symptoms, and patient satisfaction.

*Results.*—All patients who underwent dermis fat spacer grafting during lower eyelid malposition repair, noted improvement in ocular surface symptoms and restoration of normal eyelid position.

*Conclusions.*—Dermis fat is a novel posterior lamellar spacer graft and offers numerous advantages over conventional lower eyelid spacer grafts for repair of lower eyelid malposition (Figs 1, 3 and 4).

▶ In general, a diagnosis of the origin of the problem, as in all aesthetic surgeries, paramount in eyelid retraction and/or ectropion, is the problem in the skin, the lamella, the lax ligaments, or all 3. Ophthalmologists generally prefer the nuclear option and use a spacer, which will correct all of the problems with 1 operation, except severe skin deficiencies. This has great appeal; however, it is not necessary in all cases. Tightening the ligaments, alone, or tightening the ligaments in the mid face advancement may accomplish the same. If it is a hematoma of the middle lamella, which I do think causes this severe scarring and retraction without loss of tissue, does not improve in 3 months, a spacer may be necessary. However, if the conjunctivae are not

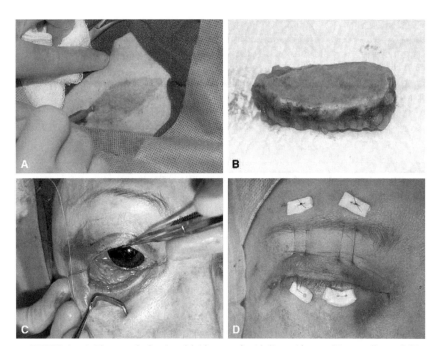

FIGURE 1.—A, Photograph showing debridement of epithelium. After marking an ellipse of skin, a high-speed diamond tip burr is used to remove the epithelial surface. Debridement continues until a fine hyperemia of the underlying dermis is noted. B, Photograph showing gross appearance of dermis fat graft. The graft is initially oversized because of shrinkage after harvesting and is contoured in situ. C, Photograph showing placement of dermis fat graft into inferior fornix. The graft is oriented with dermis side toward the ocular surface and the fat side directed anteriorly. The graft then is secured to the cut edges of the conjunctiva with interrupted sutures deep in the fornix. D, Photograph showing temporary closure of eyelid. Frost sutures are used to immobilize the eyelid for 1 week after surgery. Two 5-0 polypropylene sutures are passed from the lower tarsus and through the upper tarsus and fixated above the brow on foam bolsters. (Reprinted from Korn BS, Kikkawa DO, Cohen SR, et al. Treatment of lower eyelid malposition with dermis fat grafting. *Ophthalmology.* 2008;115:744.e2-751.e2, with permission from the American Academy of Ophthalmology.)

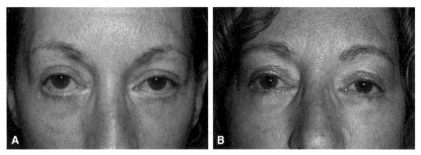

FIGURE 3.—A, Preoperative photograph of case 2 showing marked bilateral lower eyelid retraction. B, Postoperative photograph of case 2 obtained after sequential dermis fat grafting and midface elevation showing a return of normal lower eyelid position. (Reprinted from Korn BS, Kikkawa DO, Cohen SR, et al. Treatment of lower eyelid malposition with dermis fat grafting. *Ophthalmology.* 2008;115:744.e2-751.e2, with permission from the American Academy of Ophthalmology.)

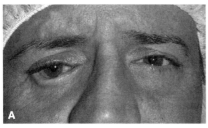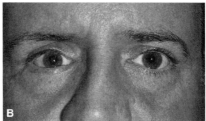

FIGURE 4.—**A,** Preoperative photograph of case 5 showing that the patient has cicatricial right lower eyelid retraction, entropion, and hypoglobus. **B,** Postoperative photograph of case 5 obtained after mid-face lifting, oversized dermis fat grafting, and lower eyelid tightening showing marked improvement. (Reprinted from Korn BS, Kikkawa DO, Cohen SR, et al. Treatment of lower eyelid malposition with dermis fat grafting. *Ophthalmology.* 2008;115:744.e2-751.e2, with permission from the American Academy of Ophthalmology.)

involved, why add this ingredient? Regrowth of hair is not enough to judge in a 1-year period, and the authors infer that there are hair follicles in the deep portion of the epidermis, which I have never seen. The follicles are in the dermis and, therefore, it takes a deep abrasion, or shaving, to remove these. In addition, the issue of ectropion versus scleral show is an important one and helps, when based on clinical experience, to make the diagnosis of what type of correction will be helpful.

**P. W. McKinney, MD, CM**

## Prevention of Lower Eyelid Malposition After Blepharoplasty: Anatomic and Technical Considerations of the Inside-Out Blepharoplasty

Rosenberg DB, Lattman J, Shah AR (Manhattan Eye, Ear, & Throat Hosp, NY)
*Arch Facial Plast Surg* 9:434-438, 2007

*Objective.*—To determine the position of the lower eyelid and lateral canthus after release of the lower eyelid retractors with the "inside-out technique" by measuring the marginal reflex distance 2 (MRD2) and using the lateral canthal rounding scale.

*Design.*—Retrospective analysis.

*Results.*—Of the 171 patients who underwent inside-out blepharoplasty, 78 were followed up for 3 months. Preoperative MRD2 was 0.942 pixels. Postoperatively, the modified MRD2 was 0.903. Although the score of the modified MRD2 was found to decrease postoperatively, the decrease was not statistically significant ($P < .07$). The lateral rounding scale reviewed an average preoperative score of 2.04 and a postoperative score of 1.99. There was no statistical difference between pre- and postoperative observations based on a 1-tailed $t$ test. No complications were reported.

*Conclusion.*—Using photographic analysis, the study found no difference in lateral canthal shape or MRD2 before and after surgery in patients who underwent inside-out blepharoplasty.

▶ The authors present a splendid explanation of the capsular palpebral mechanism with its functional component, which is basically an additional tendon for the inferior oblique muscle and the inferior rectus muscle, which lowers the lower lid on downward gaze. Cutting this initially allows the lower lid to elevate because of the upward pressure of the closure of the orbicularis. This was for the 3-month period of observation. The extent of the reattachment in the long-term is a question, and does this last? Even if it offers temporary protection, the patients may have an advantage in the immediate postoperative period.

**P. W. McKinney, MD, CM**

---

### Lower Blepharoplasty with Capsulopalpebral Fascia Hernia Repair for Palpebral Bags: A Long-Term Prospective Study

Parsa AA, Lye KD, Radcliffe N, et al (St. Francis Med Ctr, Trenton, NJ; Univ of Hawaii Honolulu; New York Univ School of Medicine, NY)
*Plast Reconstr Surg* 121:1387-1397, 2008

---

*Background.*—In December of 1998, the authors published a prospective study in *Plastic and Reconstructive Surgery* (102: 2459, 1998) comparing standard lower blepharoplasty with lipectomy on one side and fat-preserving capsulopalpebral fascia hernia repair on the contralateral side; comparable aesthetic outcomes were demonstrated after 6 months of follow-up. In the present study, the authors report their findings on the original patient cohort with an average follow-up of 11.3 years.

*Methods.*—From 1991 to 2007, 26 patients were identified who had previously undergone lower blepharoplasty for palpebral bags, using fat removal on one side and fat preservation on the contralateral side. These patients were evaluated, and the incidence and locations of palpebral bag recurrence, lower lid hollowing, lid malposition, and eyelid dysmobility were documented.

*Results.*—The overall recurrence rate of palpebral bags under the eyes following standard fat resection (30.8 percent) was significantly higher than for eyes following capsulopalpebral fascia hernia repair (7.7 percent) ($p = 0.043$). Recurrences of fat herniation, of generally less significance than the original preoperative status, were not found in any of the lower eyelid compartments in the former group, and only in the lateral compartment in the latter.

*Conclusions.*—At long-term follow-up, fat-preserving capsulopalpebral fascia repair for palpebral bags demonstrates superiority to standard blepharoplasty with lipectomy, with significantly lower recurrence of palpebral bags. In a small percentage of patients undergoing capsulopalpebral fascia hernia repair, limited fat resection in selected patients may eliminate hernia recurrence.

▶ I have always considered it somewhat strange and improbable that baggy lower eyelids were caused entirely by excessive fat, the removal of which would return the eyes to a youthful appearance. Although the authors present a long-term study and conclude that a capsulopalpebral fascia repair is superior to a standard fat removing blepaharoplasty, the evidence is still not entirely convincing in this very small study of 26 patients. For example, were the eyes equally baggy preoperatively? Was the choice of capsulopalpebral fascia repair and standard blepharoplasty chosen randomly? Finally, when one looks at several photos provided, recurrences were evident on both sides in some and in no sides in others. Also, the techniques were combined in some individuals (ie, capsulopalpebral fascia repair plus fat excision). Regardless, this is an approach worth considering, especially for the surgeon who finds many of his postoperative blepharoplasty patients have hollowing of the lower eyelids after standard blepharoplasty.

**S. H. Miller, MD, MPH**

---

**Transconjunctival Septal Suture Repair for Lower Lid Blepharoplasty**
Sadove RC (Univ of Florida, Gainesville)
*Plast Reconstr Surg* 120:521-529, 2007

---

*Background.*—The need for a safer lower-lid blepharoplasty procedure than the classic subciliary approach has long been recognized. In 1996, de la Plaza and de la Cruz first theorized septal suturing via a transconjunctival approach that preserves both muscle and infraorbital fat. This is the first report of a series of patients treated with this technique. The transconjunctival approach can avoid the complications of "scleral show" and changes in the shape of the aperture that are associated with the subciliary/muscle cutting approach to the fat pads.

*Methods.*—Transconjunctival septal suturing of the middle and medial fat bags was used to treat 78 consecutive patients (72 women and six men) with visible bulging fat of the lower eyelids. Some patients underwent simultaneous resection of fat from the lateral pad.

*Results.*—Bulging fat in the middle and medial compartments was eliminated without overtreatment or undertreatment. Substantial, but not total improvement, in tear trough deformity was often observed. Aperture shape and lid level were preserved.

*Conclusions.*—The results, achieved with this series of patients, indicate that transconjunctival suture repair of the orbital septum is a safe, predictable, and effective treatment for bulging fat of the medial and middle fat pads of the lower eyelid. Changes in aperture shape and lid level can be avoided without the need for simultaneous lid-tightening procedures.

▶ The septal repair (de la Plaza) returns fat to the eye socket and prevents the long-term hollowing of the upper lid and the lower lid. This technique, however, risks too much fat remaining in some patients. Often, a combination of extraction, laterally, repair centrally, and repositioning medially to fill the nasojugal groove is very effective.

**P. W. McKinney, MD, CM**

---

**Bipolar Coagulation-Assisted Orbital (BICO) Septoblepharoplasty: A Retrospective Analysis of a New Fat-Saving Upper-Eyelid Blepharoplasty Technique**
van der Lei B, Timmerman ISK, Cromheecke M, et al (Med Centre of Leeuwarden, The Netherlands; Erasmus Med Ctr, Rotterdam, The Netherlands)
*Ann Plast Surg* 59:263-267, 2007

---

*Background.*—Upper eyelid blepharoplasty, generally, is performed as a combination of excess skin reduction and fat resection. Fat resection can, in the long term, result in a hollow orbit. Therefore, treatment of the lax orbital septum, in combination with skin reduction, seems a more preferable approach than fat resection.

The authors describe a technique of upper-eyelid blepharoplasty: a combination of excess skin reduction and shortening of the stretched lax orbital septum by means of bipolar coagulation. This procedure is called *bi*polar coagulation-assisted *or*bital septoblepharoplasty, ie, BICO septoblepharoplasty. The aim of this retrospective study is to report on our initial experience with this technique.

*Methods.*—We retrospectively analyzed 296 patients in whom an upper-eyelid blepharoplasty was performed during the past 4 years using the BICO septoblepharoplasty technique: first, excess skin is removed, then a small rim of orbicularis muscle is excised to expose the bulging orbital septum, and finally, before closure of the wound, bipolar coagulation of the exposed orbital septum is performed. This results in shrinkage of the septum and, thus, in repositioning of the pseudoherniated fat pads.

*Results.*—At discharge from follow-up, which varied from 9 weeks (72% of the patients) up till 2 years after surgery (28% of the patients), in all patients, ultimately, a satisfactory result was achieved and, ultimately, all were satisfied or very satisfied with the result of the procedure. There were only 3 patients with minor complications: 1 patient with a slightly retracting scar, which resolved spontaneously, and 2 patients with slight asymmetry requiring additional skin resection.

*Conclusions.*—BICO septoblepharoplasty of the upper eyelid seems to be an effective way to treat blepharochalasia of the upper eyelid; the bipolar coagulation of the orbital septum will lead to shrinkage of the septum, thereby repositioning the prolapsing medial and central fat pads. Secondary fibrosis will reinforce the orbital septum, postoperatively.

▶ In applying the concept of fat preservation to the upper lids the authors used the cautery technique of Cook[1] rather than the sutures of De La Plaza,[2] furthermore indicating the safety of the bipolar cautery. Whatever the methods, the concept of maintaining a "full upper lid" is important for a youthful appearance. In using the De La Plaza technique in lower lids it may be necessary at times to remove a small amount of fat as well; in fact, in shaping a lower lid, repositioning the medial pocket to fill the nasojugal groove with partial resection in the De La Plaza of the central pocket and evacuation of the lateral pocket, will often achieve some outstanding results. Does cautery weaken the septum in the long run? Will there be recurrence? I hope not, because it is a wonderful method.

**P. W. McKinney, MD, CM**

*References*

1. Cook TA, Derebery J, Harrah R. Reconsideration of fat and management in lower eyelid blepharoplasty surgery. *Archives Otolaryngology.* 1984;10:521.
2. De La Plaza R, Arroyo JM. A new technique for the treatment of palpebral bags. *Plastic Reconstructive Surgery.* 1988;81:677.

---

**Laser-Assisted Blepharoplasty and Inferior Lateral Retinaculum Plication: Skin Contraction Versus Skin Traction**
Kontoes PP, Lambrinaki N, Vlachos SP (HYGEIA Hosp, Athens, Greece)
*Aesthetic Plast Surg* 31:579-585, 2007

---

Blepharoplasty is one of the most commonly performed operations in plastic surgery, especially among middle-aged patients. Ablative lasers, especially the carbon dioxide laser, assist in tissue cutting and hemostasis. These lasers also offer skin resurfacing with its unique advantages despite the prolonged downtime. The authors present their laser-assisted blepharoplasty experience and the recent addition of one simply performed, inferior lateral retinaculum plication to the procedure (single suture traction technique, SSTT). Hence, the need for laser skin resurfacing of the lower eyelid has been reduced due to the skin traction applied, avoiding the long period required for resolution of erythema and potential hyperpigmentation. Furthermore, the tightening effect on the canthal ligament offers a more youthful look to the surgically treated eye.

▶ Lifting the lower lid by tightening the ligaments will reduce some wrinkles alone. If this is sufficient for that patient, it is always preferable to resurfacing whether by chemicals or lasers because a burn is a burn, and it permanently alters the character of the skin.

**P. W. McKinney, MD, CM**

Anatomy of the Corrugator Supercilii Muscle: Part I. Corrugator Topography
Janis JE, Ghavami A, Lemmon JA, et al (Univ of Texas Southwestern Med Ctr, Dallas; Case Western Reserve Univ, Cleveland, OH)
*Plast Reconstr Surg* 120:1647-1653, 2007

*Background.*—Complete corrugator supercilii muscle resection is important for the surgical treatment of migraine headaches and may help prevent postoperative abnormalities in surgical forehead rejuvenation. Specific topographic analysis of corrugator supercilii muscle dimensions and its detailed association with the supraorbital nerve branching patterns has not been thoroughly delineated. Part I of this two-part study aims to define corrugator supercilii muscle topography with respect to external bony landmarks.

*Methods.*—Twenty-five fresh cadaver heads (50 corrugator supercilii muscles and 50 supraorbital nerves) were dissected to isolate the corrugator supercilii muscle from surrounding muscles. Standardized measurements of corrugator supercilii muscle dimensions were taken with respect to the nasion and lateral orbital rim.

*Results.*—Relative to the nasion, the most medial origin of the corrugator supercilii muscle was found at 2.9 ± 1.0 mm; the most lateral origin point, 14.0 ± 2.8 mm. The lateralmost insertion of the corrugator supercilii muscle measured 43.3 ± 2.9 mm from the nasion or 7.6 ± 2.7 mm medial to the lateral orbital rim. The most cephalic extent (apex) of the muscle was located 32.6 ± 3.1 mm cephalad to the nasion–lateral orbital rim plane and 18.0 ± 3.7 mm medial to the lateral orbital rim. There were no statistical differences noted between the right and left sides.

*Conclusions.*—The dimensions of the corrugator supercilii muscle are more extensive than previously described and can be easily delineated using fixed bony landmarks. These data may prove beneficial in performing safe, complete, and symmetric corrugator supercilii muscle resection for forehead rejuvenation and for effective decompression of the supraorbital nerve and supratrochlear nerve branches in the surgical treatment of migraine headaches.

▶ I find that sometimes thin sheets of this muscle especially in older females are hard to identify particularly when approached through the upper lid. The demonstration of the true extent of this muscle and its surface anatomical measurements will aid surgical and medical treatments. Although one can assimilate the muscle by having the patients furrow brows, it may be that these thin extensions are enough to cause residual furrowing.

**P. W. McKinney, MD, CM**

### The Anatomy of the Corrugator Supercilii Muscle: Part II. Supraorbital Nerve Branching Patterns

Janis JE, Ghavami A, Lemmon JA, et al (Univ of Texas Southwestern Med Ctr, Dallas, TX; Case Western Reserve Univ School of Med)
*Plast Reconstr Surg* 121:233-240, 2008

*Background.*—This article focuses on delineation of supraorbital nerve branching patterns relative to the corrugator muscle fibers and identifies four branching patterns that help improve understanding of the local anatomy.

*Methods.*—Twenty-five fresh cadaver heads (50 corrugator supercilii muscles and 50 supraorbital nerves) were dissected and the corrugator supercilii muscles isolated. After corrugator supercilii muscle measurement points were recorded for part I of the study, the supraorbital nerve branches were then traced from their emergence points from the orbit and dissected out to the defined topographical boundaries of the muscle. Nerve branching patterns relative to the muscle fibers were analyzed, and a classification system for branching patterns relative to the muscle was created.

*Results.*—Four types of supraorbital nerve branching patterns were found. In type I (40 percent), only the deep supraorbital nerve division sent branches that coursed directly along the undersurface of the muscle. In type II (34 percent), branches emerging directly from the superficial supraorbital nerve were found, in addition to the branches from the deep division. Type III (4 percent) included discrete branches from the superficial division, but none from the deep division. In type IV (22 percent), significant branching began more cephalad relative to the muscle and, therefore, displayed no specific relation to the muscle fibers.

*Conclusions.*—Contrary to previous reports, both the deep and superficial divisions of the supraorbital nerve are intimately associated with corrugator supercilii muscle fibers. Four supraorbital nerve branching patterns, from these divisions, were found. Potential sites of supraorbital nerve compression were identified. This more detailed, anatomical information may improve the safety and accuracy of performing complete corrugator supercilii muscle resection.

▶ The corrugator superciliaris has been modified and/or removed from approaches via the upper lid, a coronal flap, or endoscopically. The indirect approaches would put the supraorbital nerve at greater risk, in view of these studies; yet, I am unaware of any reports of permanent numbness or neuroma after corrugator resections. This must have happened somewhere. However, is this like rhytidectomy or rhinoplasty? We do not test for areas of numbness or probe for neuromas, and although, on occasion, I am curious as to the effects of the large skin flap or "open versus closed rhinoplasty" and how the numbness recedes, drawing attention to this may not be in the patient's best interest.

The author's findings should give us extra caution, especially if indirect approaches to the corrugator are used.

**P. W. McKinney, MD, CM**

---

**Transblepharoplasty Ptosis Repair: Three-Step Technique**
McCord CD, Seify H, Codner MA (Paces Plastic Surgery, Atlanta, GA; Univ of California at Irvine, Newport)
*Plast Reconstr Surg* 120:1037-1044, 2007

---

*Background.*—The ability to predict postoperative lid levels in ptosis surgery has been refined over the years, but there is no completely predictable formula with which to predict the final tension in the upper lid that determines the final upper lid level. A significant percentage of patients continue to require postoperative surgical revision. The authors studied the effectiveness of a technique for the quantitation of aponeurotic repair that is not a measured resection procedure, does not require voluntary patient cooperation, and can be performed under general anesthesia.

*Methods.*—The surgical technique involves reapproximation of specific anatomical landmarks, adjustment of upper lid level by eyelid gapping, and adjustment of upper lid tension with a spring-back test. Consecutive patient charts were reviewed retrospectively for age, sex, clinical examination, levator function, and outcomes, including revision rate and patient satisfaction. A total of 144 procedures were performed for 80 patients (64 bilateral and 16 unilateral). The series was reported for a 3-year period (2002 through 2005). The mean age was 62 years (range, 40 to 85 years). The average follow-up was 18 months. All patients had acquired adult ptosis with levator dehiscence and good levator function.

*Results.*—The criterion for surgical revision was a greater than 1-mm asymmetry between the eyelids or patient dissatisfaction. Twelve patients (15 percent) were considered to be slightly asymmetric postoperatively, but only two (2.5 percent) exceeded the criterion and required surgical revision in the early postoperative period (<1 year).

*Conclusion.*—Tarso levator surgery can be performed under general anesthesia using a three-step technique to correct ptosis with a superior predictability.

▶ Mild ptosis is very common in upper lid blepharoplasty in older patients. It is common because of dehiscence of the levator mechanism to the tarsus. Beware of the unilateral ptosis, as Hering's law comes into play, and the "normal" side may droop postoperatively. The approach the authors describe makes it easy to repair through the blepharoplasty incision.

**P. W. McKinney, MD, CM**

**Surgical Correction of Blepharoptosis Using the Levator Aponeurosis–Müller's Muscle Complex Readaptation Technique: A 15-Year Experience**
Scuderi N, Chiummariello S, Gado FD, et al (Univ of Rome La Sapienza, Italy)
*Plast Reconstr Surg* 121:71-78, 2008

*Background.*—Palpebral ptosis is defined as abnormal drooping of the upper lid, caused by partial or total reduction in levator muscle function. It may be caused by various abnormalities, both congenital and acquired. The aim of this article is to report the long-term follow-up of results obtained with the levator aponeurosis–Müller's muscle complex readaptation technique.

*Methods.*—In a clinical study, 144 eyelids (102 patients) affected by congenital or acquired blepharoptosis were treated using the levator aponeurosis–Müller's muscle complex readaptation technique. Degree of ptosis and levator function were measured preoperatively and postoperatively. All patients were followed up for 1 year, 54 of them for 3 years, 22 for 5 years, and 12 for 10 years.

*Results.*—Complete correction or mild residual ptosis was achieved in over 83 percent. All ptosis with preoperative levator function greater than 8 mm was completely corrected, whereas eyelids with poor or absent levator function showed a variable degree of postoperative correction and a statistically significant difference. Ptosis correction between eyelids with levator function greater than 8 mm or less than 8 mm was analyzed statistically using the McNemar test for paired data.

*Conclusions.*—This surgical technique is effective in both acquired and congenital ptosis. In particular, the authors obtained better results in those with fair to good (>8 mm) levator function than in those with poor or absent (≤8 mm) levator function.

▶ This report is an excellent presentation of data with a 15-year experience using a combined levator and Muller's muscle advancement for correction of ptosis. An additional benefit was the strengthening of the levator muscle in many patients. The postoperative results in patients with levator function of greater than 8 mm is "sufficient" in 100% of patients. However, those patients with levator function of less than 8 mm, only had 50 percent "sufficient" ptosis correction. Combined with levator strengthening data this is a powerful repair. The Muller's resection alone is less invasive, but is not strong enough for ptosis greater than 2 mm to 3 mm. For an aesthetic practice where mild acquired ptosis is frequently encountered, where there is greater than 8 mm of levator function, and where the Herring reflexes are checked (contralateral elevation of an eyelid in unilateral ptosis), I have employed the following approach for ptosis repair: measure levator function, degree of ptosis, and Herring's reflex. If the surgery includes an upper blepharoplasty, levator advancement is performed especially in the older patients that frequently have a dehiscence, allowing less dissection than levator–Muller's together. If a blepharoplasty is not to be performed, a Muller/conjunctival resection is done through the eversion technique for those patients with less than 3 mm of ptosis.

**P. W. McKinney, MD, CM**

---

**Levator Superioris Muscle Function in Involutional Blepharoptosis**
Pereira LS, Hwang TN, Kersten RC, et al (Univ of California San Francisco, CA; Cincinnati Eye Inst, OH)
*Am J Ophthalmol* 145:1095-1098, 2008

---

*Purpose.*—To assess the role of muscular degeneration, we evaluated the correlation between ptosis severity and levator muscle function.

*Design.*—Retrospective cohort study.

*Methods.*—The medical records of 136 patients (53 men and 83 women; mean age, 67 years) with acquired blepharoptosis were reviewed for levator function (LF), margin reflex distance (MRD), age, and gender. Multivariate linear regression was performed for statistical analysis.

*Results.*—A significant correlation ($P < .001$) was seen between MRD (mean, 1.0 + 1.0 mm; range, −3.0 to 3.0 mm) and LF (mean, 15.0 + 1.0 mm; range, 11.0 to 20.0 mm). On average, a 0.5-mm reduction in LF was observed for each 1.0-mm decrease in MRD. This was independent to other variables assessed.

*Conclusions.*—In patients with involutional blepharoptosis, a directly proportional decrease in levator function and eyelid height was observed. This may implicate an abnormality of the levator muscle itself as a contributing factor in the development of involutional blepharoptosis.

▶ This is an intriguing study raising the possibility that acquired involutional blepharoptosis may be due to muscular degenerative changes in the levator muscle itself. This is not a new concept, but good documentation and evidence is lacking. The hypothesis that acquired involutional blepharoptosis may be due to aponeurotic and muscular degeneration needs further study and needs correlation between measures of the margin reflex distance (MRD) and levator function (LF) and biopsy evidence of degenerative changes in the muscle, and should be a multi-institutionally conducted study to acquire adequate numbers of data points rapidly.

**S. H. Miller, MD, MPH**

**Beveled Approach for Revisional Surgery in Asian Blepharoplasty**
Chen WP-D (Univ of California, Los Angeles)
*Plast Reconstr Surg* 120:545-552, 2007

*Background.*—Primary Asian blepharoplasty can be performed with
trapezoidal debulking of the preaponeurotic platform via a beveled
approach along the upper incision line. This is a logical and efficient
method, safely approaching the preaponeurotic space through the orbital
septum. Junctional tissues overlying the supratarsal and pretarsal areas are
uniformly debulked, and the adhesions between the levator aponeurosis
and subcutaneous tissues follow the lid crease incision line. The complication rate is minimized by reducing the chance of producing an uneven
plane of surgical dissection.
*Technique for Primary Cases.*—Primary upper blepharoplasty is performed, then the skin, muscle, and preaponeurotic fat are reduced by excision. The preaponeurotic space is positioned inferiorly at closure, reaching
the area over the superior tarsal border. If the exposed preaponeurotic fat
was totally excised, the septum and preseptal orbicularis lie directly on the
levator aponeurosis, essentially eliminating the glide zone (preaponeurotic
space). In this case there is a deep supratarsal sulcus and poor crease
formation. If fat removal was partial or minimal, some may remain inter-
posed between the preseptal orbicularis and aponeurosis. With a beveled
approach, the upper skin edge is attached to the aponeurosis along the
superior tarsal border and the lower skin edge. The preaponeurotic
space, fat to the superior tarsal border, and fat-buffering in the glide
zone are preserved. The orbicularis is transected in an upwardly beveled
manner, removing more orbicularis fibers along the upper incision edge,
the upper incisional skin edge contacts the preaponeurotic space.
The second and third approaches preserve the preaponeurotic space
over the preseptal midregion of the upper lid. The crese formed is dynamic
and appears natural. Restoring and preserving this aponeurotic space is an
essential element in creating a lid crease for Asians with a creaseless eyelid.
The up-vectored tarsal plate and preserved fat contribute to create a well-
formed crease.
*Revision Technique.*—In revisions, the glide zone has no significant preaponeurotic fat pads in its lowest aspect. Instead, a condensed apron of
tissue limits up-vectoring of the posterior layer to lie against passive, flexible skin or orbicularis. Crease formation is nonexistent and the patient
often reports fatigue, tightness, and overaction of the brow and forehead.
The incision in these cases must not add to the scarred field of operation
either esthetically or functionally.
The revision technique is initially similar to a primary approach but the
upper and lower lines of incisions are directly next to each other on either
side of the existing incisional scar on the upper eyelid. A full-thickness skin
incision is made along the marked lines, then sharp-tipped spring scissors
are used to incise across the upper incision line in a beveled fashion, with
skin-to-orbicularis adhesions. The scissoring motions remain small in

transecting the middle lamella scar after traversing the fasical layers between the orbicularis and levator aponeurosis. The beveled approach is steeper than in primary cases. The preaponeurotic fat pad will not be as large. After the forehead/eyebrow/preseptal skin layer are carefully reset, the scarred tissues of the anterior layer and midlamellar zone are excised but the remaining skin must permit passive eyelid closure, fat is preserved. A gentle downward pull on the tarsal plate will show any objective restrictions of movement; asking the patient to gaze up and down will assess subjective restrictions.

Using the superiorly beveled approach partially restores the glide space and removes scarring. Interfering tissues are removed from the preaponeurotic platform. Residual fat pads in the glide zone can fill in the space as appropriate. The skin above the incision can now form a contrasting eyelid fold.

*Conclusion.*—Revisional blepharoplasty in Asian subjects can be accomplished with a superiorly beveled approach. This restores the glide zone, removes the middle lamellar scar, and eliminates interfering tissues from the preaponeurotic platform. In many cases, an abnormally high, static scar can be repositioned into a lower, more natural, and dynamic crease without the need for skin grafting.

▶ Beveling superiorly resects an unequal wedge; therefore, more scar and fat superiorly, which will accentuate the crease. The emphasis on 'natural' is important, as when Asian blepharoplasty became popular after World War II, the result had a distinctive Caucasian appearance partially generated by an American's wish and partially generated by surgeon inexperience. Today's emphasis is on ethnic identity and to me is more harmonious.

**P. W. McKinney, MD, CM**

---

### Superior Oblique Tendon Damage Resulting from Eyelid Surgery
Kushner BJ, Jethani JN (Univ of Wisconsin, Madison)
*Am J Ophthalmol* 144:943-948, 2007

---

*Purpose.*—To describe the occurrence of superior oblique (SO) tendon damage resulting from upper eyelid surgery and to explain its cause and treatment.

*Design.*—Retrospective, observational case series.

*Methods.*—An institution-based retrospective observational case series of seven patients in whom damage to the SO tendon secondary to eyelid surgery developed.

*Results.*—In four of the patients, ipsilateral SO palsy developed, and three patients, a Brown syndrome pattern developed. The causative eyelid procedures consisted of surgery to correct ptosis in four patients, tumor removal in two patients, and cosmetic blepharoplasty in one patient.

*Conclusions.*—The SO tendon may be damaged as a result of eyelid surgery. The anatomy of the SO tendon should be kept in mind while performing surgery in the superomedial aspect of the upper eyelid.

▶ We have no statistics regarding incidents of this complication, which fortunately appears to be rare, but it is an extremely important problem when surgery is done in the region of the medial aspect of the upper lids even occurring in seemingly safe procedures, such as blepharoplasty and levator resections. Damage to the superior oblique tendon affects the inward and upward motion of the eye. A neutral position appearance will not be changed.

**P. W. McKinney, MD, CM**

## Face, Neck, and Brow

### The dynamic rotation of Langer's lines on facial expression
Bush J, Ferguson MWJ, Mason T, et al (Renovo plc, Manchester, England; Univ of Manchester, England)
*J Plast Reconstr Aesthetic Surg* 60:393-399, 2007

Karl Langer investigated directional variations in the mechanical and physical properties of skin [Gibson T. Editorial. Karl Langer (1819–1887) and his lines. *Br J Plast Surg* 1978; **31**:1–2]. He produced a series of diagrams depicting lines of cleavage in the skin [Langer K. On the anatomy and physiology of the skin I. The cleavability of the cutis. *Br J Plast Surg* 1978; **31**:3–8] and showed that the orientation of these lines coincided with the dominant axis of mechanical tension in the skin [Langer K. On the anatomy and physiology of the skin II. Skin tension. *Br J Plast Surg* 1978; **31**:93–106]. Previously, these lines have been considered as a static feature. We set out to determine whether Langer's lines have a dynamic element and to define any rotation of the orientation of Langer's lines on the face with facial movement.

One hundred and seventy-five naevi were excised from the face and neck of 72 volunteers using circular dermal punch biopsies. Prior to surgery, a vertical line was marked on the skin through the centre of each naevus. After excision, distortions of the resulting wounds were observed. The orientation of the long axis of each wound, in relation to the previously marked vertical line, was measured with a goniometer with the volunteer at rest and holding their face in five standardised facial expressions: mouth open, smiling, eyes tightly shut, frowning and eyebrows raised. The aim was to measure the orientation of the long axis of the wound with the face at rest and subsequent rotation of the wound with facial movement.

After excision, elliptical distortion was seen in 171 of the 175 wounds at rest. Twenty-nine wounds maintained the same orientation of distortion in all of the facial expressions. In the remaining wounds, the long axis of the wound rotated by up to 90°. The amount of rotation varied between sites ($p > 0.0001$).

We conclude that Langer's lines are not a static feature but are dynamic, with rotation of up to 90°. It is possible that this rotation in the axis of mechanical tension will affect the appearance of the resulting scar.

▶ Right angles to the direction of major muscle pull gives the least scar, rather than relying upon Langer's lines. This appears to be what is occurring in these patients. Inherent skin tension, which Langer measures, is interesting, but not as powerful a force as the muscle creasing.

**P. W. McKinney, MD, CM**

---

### The Fat Compartments of the Face: Anatomy and Clinical Implications for Cosmetic Surgery

Rohrich RJ, Pessa JE (Univ of Texas Southwestern Med Ctr, Dallas)
*Plast Reconstr Surg* 119:2219-2227, 2007

---

*Background.*—Observation suggests that the subcutaneous fat of the face is partitioned as distinct anatomical compartments.

*Methods.*—Thirty hemifacial cadaver dissections were performed after methylene blue had been injected into specified regions. Initial work focused on the nasolabial fat. Dye was allowed to set for a minimum of 24 hours to achieve consistent diffusion. Dissection was performed in the cadaver laboratory using microscopic and loupe magnification.

*Results.*—The subcutaneous fat of the face is partitioned into multiple, independent anatomical compartments. The nasolabial fold is a discrete unit with distinct anatomical boundaries. What has been referred to as malar fat is composed of three separate compartments: medial, middle, and lateral temporal-cheek fat. The forehead is similarly composed of three anatomical units including central, middle, and lateral temporal-cheek fat. Orbital fat is noted in three compartments determined by septal borders. Jowl fat is the most inferior of the subcutaneous fat compartments. Some of the structures, referred to as "retaining ligaments", are formed, simply, by fusion points of abutting septal barriers of these compartments.

*Conclusions.*—The subcutaneous fat of the face is partitioned into discrete anatomic compartments. Facial aging is, in part, characterized by how these compartments change with age. The concept of separate compartments of fat suggests that the face does not age as a confluent or composite mass. Shearing between adjacent compartments may be an additional factor in the etiology of soft-tissue malposition. Knowledge of this anatomy will lead to better understanding, and greater precision, in the preoperative analysis and surgical treatment of the aging face.

▶ The fusion points of the individual fat compartments may make up retaining ligaments, and these ligaments attach to the deeper structures, such as the periosteum, as Stuzin and I believe (see discussion by James Stuzin). Does releasing these in the sub-SMAS plane of a facelift flatten the face by compressing these fat compartments, and is this particularly true in repeated lifts, flattening the facial appearance?

**P. W. McKinney, MD, CM**

---

**Botulinum Toxin A for Lower Facial Contouring: A Prospective Study**
Yu C-C, Chen PK-T, Chen Y-R (Chang Gung Univ, Gueihsan, Taiwan)
*Aesthetic Plast Surg* 31:445-451, 2007

---

*Background.*—A prominent mandibular angle is a common reason for aesthetic treatment among Asian women. Such women usually present with hypertrophic masseteric muscles, and one treatment for this uses botulinum toxin A (BoNTA). Detailed effectiveness and physiologic influences of this therapy are still under investigation.

*Methods.*—The authors report a prospective study of 10 female volunteers with hypertrophic masseteric muscles who received a single treatment comprising intramuscular injection of BoNTA. The facial change and the discomfort of the injection were self-rated using a visual analog scale, and the patients were regularly inspected up to 1 year. Bite forces also were measured for chronological documentation. Volume changes of masticating muscles were evaluated by three-dimensional computed tomography (CT) scans before and 3 months after injection of BoNTA.

*Results.*—The serial photographs and patient subjective evaluation showed an obvious facial change 3 to 6 months after injection. Bite forces decreased from the first day after injection, but started to recover during week 3 and were normal 3 months after injection. Three-dimensional CT evaluation showed a statistically significant mean masseter reduction of about 30%, but no change in the volume of other masticating muscles. There were no serious complications during this study.

*Conclusions.*—Injection of BoNTA is an effective alternative for contouring of the lower facial profile by reducing the bulkiness of masseteric muscles. Its effectiveness was noticed as early as 2 weeks after injection and reached a peak effect in month 3. The facial contour gradually returned 6 months after injection. The reduction in bite force was temporary and caused no daily life interference.

▶ In Dr Michael Kane's discussion of this article[1] he brings up many good points concerning the mechanism of action of Botox especially in the debate as to whether it is muscle atrophy or muscle compensation for the temporarily paralyzed portion. For example, the quick results in denervation of the depressor angularis oris may be a compensatory factor rather than the paresis.

**P. W. McKinney, MD, CM**

*Reference*

    1. Kane MA. Botulinum toxin a for lower facial contouring: a prospective study. Discussion. *Aesthetic Plast Surg.* 2007;31:452-453.

## The Face Recurve Concept: Medical and Surgical Applications

Le Louarn C, Buthiau D, Buis J (Clinique Spontini, Paris; Institut de Radiologie de Paris)
*Aesthetic Plast Surg* 31:219-231, 2007

    The application of the Face Recurve theory gives rise to new technical opportunities in the fields of both aesthetic medicine and aesthetic surgery to block the action of the age marker fascicules largely responsible for aging of the paramedian folds. With respect to aesthetic medicine, the combination of botulinum toxin and soft tissue fillers has proven effective. On the basis of the authors' theory, however, two new technical refinements become pertinent. First, the filler must be injected predominantly deep to the muscle to treat the skin depressions in a more natural manner, bringing restoration to the curve of the overlying muscle. Second, a very low number of botulinum toxin units (one-fourth to one unit) should be injected into specific muscles to diminish their resting tone without diminishing their maximal contraction strength. With respect to aesthetic surgery, the authors present new techniques for the treatment of early aging, specifically, a combination of segmental muscular section, microliposuction, and retromuscular fat grafting, all of which can be performed

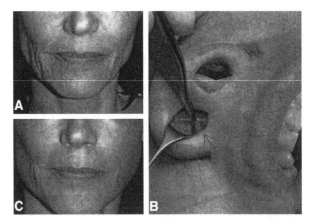

FIGURE 3.—(A) A patient with a hollow superior nasolabial sulcus and elevated ala because of the high resting tone of the levator alaeque nasi muscle. The nasal ala is depressed against the pyriform aperture. (B) An intercartilaginous approach. At this point, the levator alaeque nasi muscle is seen close to bone. (C) After surgical section of the levator alaeque nasi muscle and injection of fat 0.7 ml over the pyriform aperture, the ala has descended, and depression of the upper nasolabial sulcus has diminished. (Courtesy of Le Louarn C, Buthiau D, Buis J. The face recurve concept: medical and surgical applications. *Aesthetic Plast Surg.* 2007, 31:219-231, with permission from Springer Science+Business Media, LLC.)

readily with the patient under local anesthesia. For more advanced aging, surgery offers new treatment opportunities that include the concentric malar lift for correction of the midface region, with repositioning of suborbicularis oculi fat back onto the orbital rim from its descended eccentric displacement at the hands of repeated orbicularis oculi contractions. At the same time, specific muscles can be weakened and fat volume restored. Each area can be studied in a specific way and treated definitively. Currently, the skin does not need to be tensioned to a maximum during a face-lift for treatment of the irregular jaw line, the palpebromalar groove, and so forth. Skin tension can be moderated to remove only the true excess of skin. Facial contour is improved, whereas the specific glide is restored between muscles and their underlying fat (Fig 3).

▶ The selective sectioning of facial muscles for facial rejuvenation began with Skoog 40 years ago and was also used for hyperactive muscles in facial paralysis, but this technique can leave depressions in thin skin coverage and motor nerve damage. This was particularly true in Skoog's orbicularis oculi sectioning. The choice of Botox makes these latter problems temporary. Weakening the levator alaeque nasi is particularly useful for the medial part of the nasolabial fold, which is a particularly refractory area.

**P. W. McKinney, MD, CM**

---

### Chin Surgery IV: The Large Chin—Key Parameters for Successful Chin Reduction

Zide BM, Warren SM, Spector JA (New York Univ; Cornell Univ, NY)
*Plast Reconstr Surg* 120:630 537, 2007

---

*Background.*—Treatment of macrogenia can be a challenging problem. In this article, the authors provide novel insights for treatment of a previously poorly treated problem. The authors have developed anatomical insights that facilitate the subtly difficult preoperative evaluation of the large chin and, when applied appropriately, will provide uniformly pleasing results.

*Methods.*—A retrospective review of the senior author's (B.M.Z.) patient records was performed. More than 50 cases of macrogenia were identified. As previously described, almost all of the cases were performed under local anesthesia with oral premedication only.

*Results.*—This article demonstrates why prior modalities, such as intraoral burring and lower border setback, failed to treat the variety of large chins properly. The nine critical factors the surgeon must consider in developing a successful surgical plan are outlined. The surgical plan is not primarily based on radiographs as much as on direct tactile and visual analysis of the sublabial structures both in repose and while smiling. Crucial aspects of the operative technique are highlighted.

*Conclusions.*—The large chin can be approached with confidence if nine parameters are appreciated. The authors have outlined these key variables that facilitate proper preoperative topographic analysis of the large chin. Once these variables are appreciated, an appropriate surgical plan can be formulated.

▶ Chin 'reductions' are more problematical than augmentation, which, in themselves, can be difficult. The authors emphasize the soft tissue contributions and the bony component of hypertrophy. Note the subtle changes in this surgery.

**P. W. McKinney, MD, CM**

## Chin Surgery V: Treatment of the Long, Nonprojecting Chin
Warren SM, Spector JA, Zide BM (New York Univ)
*Plast Reconstr Surg* 120:760-768, 2007

*Background.*—Correction of the long, nonprojecting chin requires both vertical reduction and sagittal augmentation. Wedge excision-based therapy reduces chin height and allows for advancement of the distal segment, but it is associated with at least a 10 percent incidence of mental nerve injury. The authors propose two innovative ways to correct the long, nonprojecting chin.

*Methods.*—There are two approaches, intraoral and extraoral. With the intraoral approach, following a gingivobuccal incision, a single horizontally oblique osteotomy is made at least 6 mm beneath the mental nerve foramina. The vertically long genial segment is freed and the posterior edge is contoured with a side-cutting burr. The contoured jumping genial segment is secured to the mandible with countersunk screws and contoured in situ to preserve the lower 8 to 10 mm. With the extraoral approach, following a submental incision, the anterior and posterior surfaces of the symphysis are cleared (a double-armed suture is placed through the posterior musculature). A reciprocating saw is used to remove the lower border of the symphysis to reduce the vertical excess. The tagged musculature is resuspended, and a tapered, textured implant is secured to the new symphysis.

*Results.*—Aesthetic outcomes using these two techniques were good and there were no complications. Representative patients, operated on by the senior author, illustrate these techniques.

*Conclusions.*—Both the intraoral one-cut in situ contoured jumping genioplasty and the extraoral vertical reduction/sagittal augmentation genioplasty reduce excess chin height, control sagittal advancement, provide pogonion projection, and avoid the risks of a standard wedge.

Both techniques provide custom projection at the lower pole of the new symphysis.

▶ The authors make a strong point that cutting bone 6 mm below the foramen will avoid damage to the nerve. If 6 mm is not available, resuspension of the muscles and a porous fixed implant (because of the extent of dissection) is required. Otherwise, advancement on an angle of the bony fragment fixes the muscle, advances the chin, and shortens the height.

**P. W. McKinney, MD, CM**

---

**Chin Surgery VI: Treatment of an Unusual Deformity, the Tethered Microgenic Chin**
Spector JA, Warren SM, Zide BM (New York Univ)
*Plast Reconstr Surg* 120:1053-1059, 2007

---

*Background.*—Although the condition is rare, some children are born with cervical clefts or masses that require repair during infancy. The scarring in the submental region can tether the developing mandible at the menton, producing a developmental microgenia or "tethered chin."
*Methods.*—A retrospective review of the senior author's (B.M.Z.) patient records was performed; three cases of tethered chin were identified. In each case, a staged surgical approach was used.
*Results.*—In two cases, previous unsuccessful surgery complicated the initial presentation. In all cases, the underlying soft-tissue anomalies were addressed and the microgenia was corrected. Satisfactory aesthetic and functional results were obtained.
*Conclusions.*—The tethered chin represents a rare entity. Correction of the tethered chin requires a comprehensive understanding of the underlying abnormality and an appreciation of the multiple factors that contribute to chin function and aesthetics.

▶ The correction of soft tissue bands is a key component of this surgery and must be planned to avoid neck scars. The authors inherited these cases, so the external scars were preordained. In the first instance, subcutaneous dissection and/or expansion of neck skin if tight could avoid these scars if the transverse incisions in skin creases are used. If the subcutaneous scarring involves the dermis then, of course, there is no alternative. An incision requiring a Z is always going to be prominent in a young individual.

**P. W. McKinney, MD, CM**

## Chin Surgery VII: The Textured Secured Implant—A Recipe for Success
Warren SM, Spector JA, Zide BM (New York Univ)
*Plast Reconstr Surg* 120:1378-1385, 2007

*Background.*—Silicone chin augmentation remains a popular treatment for microgenia because its placement appears deceptively simple. However, when extrusion, displacement, capsular contracture following implant removal, overaugmentation, or malposition occurs, a revision operation may be required. Secondary chin surgery is challenging because (1) implant removal alone may produce a disfigured chin; and (2) placement of a new implant in an oversized misshapen pocket demands precision, control, and reliability.

*Methods.*—The textured implant may be placed by means of an intraoral or extraoral route. The extraoral route is usually chosen except when transoral procedures (e.g., mentalis suspension) are required. The superior 30 to 50 percent of a standard textured implant is always removed and then tapered anteriorly at a 45-degree angle to reduce its sharp front edge. The lateral wings are also reduced and tapered. Two pilot holes are drilled in each half of the implant and then it is divided in the midline. Each half is inserted and secured individually. The medial screw is placed first and nearly fully tightened. Then, holding the implant exactly along the inferior border of the mandible, the distal screw is placed and both screws are tightened completely. The lower border of the implant should be *exactly* along the lower border of the mandible. The soft tissues are closed in three layers over a drain.

*Results.*—This technique has been used to treat more than 100 patients. Selected photographs illustrate this technique.

*Conclusion.*—This article explains how to place a textured implant efficiently and effectively under light premedication and local anesthesia.

▶ The 'texture' is really a porous implant allowing tissue ingrowth, which the authors suggest may prevent chin ptosis. Intraoral incisions have increased complication rates (infection, displacement, and muscle instability) and are usually not necessary, as a small submental incision does not show. The authors further argue that fixation and custom trim have lower complication rates. Custom trimming, of course, is easier in the textured porous implants. The negative tissue ingrowth is removal of the implant if necessary because of the tissue ingrowth. A smooth implant with 2 mm holes interspaced will allow tissue fixation with less to dissect in the unusual event of needing removal, and it works well in the smaller less complicated cases with minimal dissection. Maximal dissection, such as shown by these authors, will require a screw fixation.

**P. W. McKinney, MD, CM**

### Doppler Ultrasound Evaluation of Facial Transverse and Infraorbital Arteries: Influence of Smoking and Aging Process

Jacobovicz J, Tolazzi AR, Timi JR (Federal Univ of Parana, Brazil)
*Aesthetic Plast Surg* 31:526-531, 2007

*Background.*—Plastic surgeons are always concerned about integrity of facial vascularization in smokers and elderly candidates for face-lifting. Using Doppler ultrasound, this study aimed to evaluate influence of chronic smoking and aging on facial transverse and infraorbital artery blood flow.

*Methods.*—For this study, 40 healthy volunteer women were submitted to bilateral Doppler ultrasound of facial transverse and infraorbital arteries. Volunteers were divided into three groups: group 1 (13 nonsmoking women ages 18–33 years), group 2 (13 nonsmoking women ages 55–70 years), and group 3 (14 smoking women ages 55–70 years). Blood flow parameters measured were peak systolic velocity, end-diastolic velocity, resistivity index, and pulsatility index.

*Results.*—Chronic smoking did not cause statistically significant alterations in peak systolic velocity in any of the arteries. However, there was a significant augmentation of end-diastolic velocity and a reduction in resistivity and pulsatility index in both arteries. Aging process did not significantly alter any of the parameters evaluated. Findings in both sides of the face were similar for both arteries.

*Conclusions.*—Chronic smoking significantly altered end-diastolic velocity, resistivity, and pulsatility index in regional arterial circulation of the face. Aging process, however, did not significantly influence any of blood flow parameters studied.

▶ Here is more evidence of the negative effects of tobacco use on the circulation and its potential for increasing the complications in elective surgery. But what of cessation of tobacco use before surgery? How long is this necessary? There is evidence that some of this vasoconstriction is reversed in abstinence, but there is chronic damage as well. With experience, operations for smokers can be done, but the surgical procedures must be modified depending upon the pre- and intra-operative judgment of the vascular conditions. In face-lift patients, for example, if there are any changes in the flap, the amount of undermining must be severely limited, and tension has to be adjusted accordingly. A different type of facelift can be done—one with less skin undermining and a deeper plane. Of course, explaining this to the patient ahead of time will help them to understand the difficulties and why a compromise may be indicated.

**P. W. McKinney, MD, CM**

**Outcome Measures in Facial Plastic Surgery Patient-Reported and Clinical Efficacy Measures**
Rhee JS, McMullin BT (Med College of Wisconsin, WI; Zablocki Veteran Affairs Med Ctr, Milwaukee)
*Arch Facial Plast Surg* 10:194-207, 2008

*Objective.*—To survey the existing literature to identify, summarize, and evaluate procedure- and condition-specific outcome measures for use in facial plastic and reconstructive surgery.

*Methods.*—A review of the English-language literature was performed to identify outcomes instruments specific for targeted facial plastic surgery interventions and conditions. A search was performed using MEDLINE (1950 to September 2007), CINAHL (Cumulative Index to Nursing & Allied Health) (1982 to September 2007), and PsychINFO (1806 to September 2007). Outcomes instruments were categorized as patient-reported or clinical efficacy measures (observer-reported or objective measures). Instruments were then categorized to include relevant details on the intervention, degree of validation, and subsequent use.

*Results.*—Sixty-eight distinct instruments were identified (23 patient-reported, 35 observer-reported, and 10 objective measures), with some overlap among categories. Most patient-reported measures (76%) and half observer-reported instruments (51%) were developed in the past 10 years. The rigor of validation varied widely among measures, with formal validation being most common among the patient-reported outcome measures.

*Conclusions.*—Validated outcomes measures are present for many common facial plastic surgery conditions and have become more prevalent during the past decade, especially for patient-reported outcomes. Challenges remain in harmonizing patient-reported, observer-based, and other objective measures to produce standardized clinically meaningful outcome measures.

▶ There is little question that as a generalization in the 21st Century, reliable, valid, and inexpensive measurement tools are needed to assess outcomes and provide data, which leads to evidence-based medical practice. It is evident that these principles must apply, not only to heart surgery, management of diabetes etc, but also equally to plastic surgical practice including facial plastic surgery. This study clearly shows that there are, in fact, multiple outcome measures (patient-centered, expert evaluation, and objective measures) to assess the results of facial plastic surgery, but little in the way of agreement as to which should be used, by whom and when. In my view, the only way to bring clarity and rationality to this area of medical practice is to establish study collaboratives; collaboratives where the participant surgeons agree on inclusion/exclusion criteria for patients having surgery, which measurement tool(s) to use and when to assess the results. It is only through such collaboratives, that plastic surgeons will be able to measure their results against generally accepted outcome standards and use that information for improvement. It will also potentially provide patients the opportunity to base their decisions regarding surgeons on normative standards.

S. H. Miller, MD, MPH

## Experience with Fibrin Glue in Rhytidectomy
Kamer FM, Nguyen DB (Lasky Clinic, Beverly Hills, CA; Univ of Southern California, Los Angeles; Univ of California, Los Angeles)
*Plast Reconstr Surg* 120:1045-1051, 2007

*Background.*—The authors conducted a large, prospective, controlled trial of fibrin glue in rhytidectomy using a wide set of variables.

*Methods.*—Two hundred consecutive patients undergoing elective rhytidectomy were studied. One hundred patients received fibrin glue over a 1-year period and were followed prospectively. Another 100 patients from the previous year who had not received fibrin glue had their charts reviewed retrospectively. All patients underwent bilateral face lifts using the deep plane technique.

*Results.*—The following data were observed for the glue versus nonglue patients: expanding hematoma rate, 1 percent versus 3 percent ($p > 0.05$); seroma rate, 1 percent versus 7 percent ($p > 0.05$); and prolonged induration, edema, and ecchymosis, 0 percent versus 22 percent ($p < 0.05$). The pain score for glue versus nonglue patients was 100 percent minimal versus 95 percent minimal and 5 percent moderate ($p > 0.05$). The average score for patient satisfaction (scale, 1 to 10, with 10 being best) for glue versus nonglue patients was 9.5 versus 9.0 ($p > 0.05$).

*Conclusions.*—The use of fibrin glue was associated with some benefits for rhytidectomy. Fibrin glue eliminated the use of drains. The difference in expanding hematoma was clinically, but not statistically, significant. The seroma rate was decreased and neared statistical significance. There was an impressive immediate decrease in postoperative swelling. The fibrin glue was most advantageous in eliminating prolonged induration, edema, and ecchymosis. There were no statistical differences between groups for patient satisfaction or pain. The use of fibrin glue has been shown to reduce some of the morbidity and severe complications of face lifting.

▶ A loose subcutaneous suture (4 to 5) obviates the need for drains, which is a closure I learned from Hans Brook. I do not use fibrin glue because of my concern with the blood products. The loose closure and a pressure dressing allow drainage through the edges and gives in many cases a superior scar to that of multiple skin sutures with both putting them in and taking them out having caused trauma.

P. W. McKinney, MD, CM

## The Efficacy of Surgical Drainage in Cervicofacial Rhytidectomy: A Prospective, Randomized, Controlled Trial

Jones BM, Grover R, Hamilton S (King Edward VII's Hosp Sister Agnes, London)
*Plast Reconstr Surg* 120:263-270, 2007

*Background.*—Postoperative drainage is often used instinctively in face lifting with the assumption that it may reduce the likelihood of complications. This potential benefit should be balanced against cost, discomfort, and the possibility of provoking bleeding and hematoma on removal. Evidence-based decisions on drainage are problematic, since no prospective studies have examined its role. This study was designed to address this issue directly.

*Methods.*—Fifty consecutive patients undergoing face lift over a 3-month period were randomized to drainage of one side of the face only, with the contralateral side serving as a paired control. Bruising, swelling, and hematoma or seroma were assessed objectively, independently of the operating surgeon and subjectively by the patients.

*Results.*—Postoperative hematoma and edema were not influenced by the use of drains ($p > 0.5$). Patients reported no difference between the two sides, with respect to swelling ($p = 0.6$) or discomfort ($p = 0.5$). However, drains produced a statistically significant reduction in postoperative bruising both on clinical assessment ($p = 0.005$) and patient assessment ($p = 0.002$).

*Conclusions.*—This article represents the first prospective, randomized, controlled trial, assessing the use of postoperative drainage in facial rejuvenation surgery. Surgical drains do not influence postoperative complications, but they do significantly reduce bruising and may facilitate the patient's return to normal activity.

► It would have been useful to know the intraoperative and recovery room blood pressures. Controlling this has a major role in bleeding during, and immediately, after rhytidectomy. It is also important to know the type of closure performed. For example, a loose minimal stitch closure allows blood to drain itself. For example, a temple to occiput incision can be closed with less scarring with 3-4 subcutaneous dissolvable sutures and no cutaneous sutures. The latter are traumatic to place and to remove. There is less trauma to the wound edge, and the openings allow for drainage. As one gains experience with surgery, one tends to use less sutures, not out of impatience, but for a better end result. Many "petit point" 6-0 sutures, which we are taught is a good closure when we are young, is really more traumatic.

**P. W. McKinney, MD, CM**

### A Comparison of Face Lift Techniques in Eight Consecutive Sets of Identical Twins

Antell DE, Orseck MJ (Manhattan Eye, Ear and Throat Hosp, NY)

*Plast Reconstr Surg* 120:1667-1673, 2007

*Background.*—Selecting the "correct" face lift technique has always been a difficult decision for the plastic surgeon. A technique that provides optimal aesthetics for one patient may not provide the same result for another. The complexity of comparing these different results on patients with different facial features further confounds one's ability to decide on a given technique. Even identical twins are often treated more appropriately with a different technique from one twin to the other because the character and severity of facial aging may differ between them. By comparing different superficial musculoaponeurotic system techniques on "less different" people (identical twins), perhaps the ideal technique may be determined.

*Methods.*—Between November of 1997 and April of 1999, eight sets of twins underwent face lift surgery by the senior author (D.E.A.), using one of four techniques. The charts and photographs of the eight consecutive pairs of twins (16 patients) were reviewed retrospectively.

*Results.*—No one face lift technique performed in this study produced a superior result as compared with another when performed on the appropriate patient.

*Conclusion.*—There exists no face lift technique suitable for every patient. As the current literature suggests, there is no one "best" face lift technique of those studied.

▶ "Quid bene diagnoscit bene curat" is a basic pillar of medical practice (make a good diagnosis and you will make a good cure). Using twins for comparison of outcomes of surgical techniques is intriguing but flawed. Because of environmental influences, endocrine factors (eg, osteoporosis), muscle usage, and exposure to toxins, such as tobacco, all influence the tissue. Quantum sufficit (QS) is the shorthand used in prescription writing to indicate a sufficient quantity to make a certain amount. I use it in the surgical sense to mean that you do what is necessary to correct the problem at hand. As the authors imply, a "so and so" face-lift is not applicable to all patients—even subgroups of patients—and variations are wisely done by an experienced surgeon to adjust to the tissue conditions. Labels, although convenient, may be deceptive.

**P. W. McKinney, MD, CM**

### Age-Related Changes of the Orbit and Midcheek and the Implications for Facial Rejuvenation

Mendelson BC, Hartley W, Scott M, et al (Toorak Cosmetic Surgery Centre, Australia; et al)
*Aesthet Plast Surg* 31:419-423, 2007

*Background.*—Aging of the midface is complex and poorly understood. Changes occur not only in the facial soft tissues, but also in the underlying bony structure. Computed tomography (CT) imaging was used for investigating characteristics of the bony orbit and the anterior wall of the maxilla in patients of different ages and genders.

*Methods.*—Facial CT scans were performed for 62 patients ranging in age from 21 to 70 years, who were divided into three age groups: 21–30 years, 41–50 years, and 61–70 years. Patients also were grouped by gender. The lengths of the orbital roof and floor and the angle of the anterior wall of the maxilla were recorded on parasagittal images through the midline of the orbit for each patient.

*Results.*—The lengths of the orbital roof and floor at their midpoints showed no significant differences between the age groups. When grouped by gender, the lengths were found to be statistically longer for males than for females. The angle between the anterior maxillary wall and the orbital floor was found to have a statistically significant decrease with advancing age among both sexes.

*Conclusion.*—Bony changes occur in the skeleton of the midcheek with advancing age for both males and females. The anterior maxillary wall retrudes in relation to the bony orbit, which maintains a fixed anteroposterior dimension at its midpoint. These changes should be considered in addressing the aging midface.

▶ The surgeon can observe bony changes by comparing changes in younger and older skulls in the anatomy museums, the most striking of which are in the alveoli in edentulous patients. Augmentation of these changes dramatically alters the soft tissues, a common example being the use of dentures. Subtle changes in other areas, such as a 3 mm chin implant in rhytidectomy, help with the neck, and a similar effect is gained with a cheek implant and its support of the mid face. These changes were not indicated when the patient was younger, and were, therefore, not image changing operations, which in older patients are less well tolerated. Thus, filling the skin envelope adds to the tightening of the envelope, as does the lift itself. This can be done with soft tissue fillers as well, such as fat augmentation in the malar area in conjunction with a rhytidectomy.

**P. W. McKinney, MD, CM**

**Age-Related Changes of the Orbit and Midcheek and the Implications for Facial Rejuvenation**
Mendelson BC, Hartley W, Scott M, et al (Toorak Cosmetic Surgery Centre, Victoria, Australia; Harbor-UCLA, Los Angeles)
*Aesthetic Plast Surg* 31:419-423, 2007

*Background.*—Aging of the midface is complex and poorly understood. Changes occur not only in the facial soft tissues, but also in the underlying bony structure. Computed tomography (CT) imaging was used for investigating characteristics of the bony orbit and the anterior wall of the maxilla in patients of different ages and genders.

*Methods.*—Facial CT scans were performed for 62 patients ranging in age from 21 to 70 years, who were divided into three age groups: 21–30 years, 41–50 years, and 61–70 years. Patients also were grouped by gender. The lengths of the orbital roof and floor and the angle of the anterior wall of the maxilla were recorded on parasagittal images through the midline of the orbit for each patient.

*Results.*—The lengths of the orbital roof and floor at their midpoints showed no significant differences between the age groups. When grouped by gender, the lengths were found to be statistically longer for males than for females. The angle between the anterior maxillary wall and the orbital floor was found to have a statistically significant decrease with advancing age among both sexes.

*Conclusion.*—Bony changes occur in the skeleton of the midcheek with advancing age for both males and females. The anterior maxillary wall retrudes in relation to the bony orbit, which maintains a fixed anteroposterior dimension at its midpoint. These changes should be considered in addressing the aging midface.

▶ Further proof amidst facial skeletal absorption occurs with age; but in this article, the author shows that it does not involve the orbital rims. The regression of the underlying maxilla argues for volume replacement and correction of skin laxity.

**P. W. McKinney, MD, CM**

**Reversing Brow Lifts**
Yaremchuk MJ, O'Sullivan N, Benslimane F (Harvard Med School; private practice, Casablanca, Morocco)
*Aesthetic Surg J* 27:367-375, 2007

*Background.*—Undesirable brow shape and position may occur after brow lift surgery. Problems can include overelevation of the brows, separation of the brows, and creation of an apex medial slant brow shape.

*Objective.*—We report on a procedure to restore or improve presurgical brow shape and position.

*Methods.*—Brow lift reversal surgery was performed with open approaches. Anterior and posterior scalp flaps were developed in a subperiosteal plane. The lowered medial brow was sutured to the frontal bone with an anchor system. The repositioned anterior hairline was secured in a similar manner. The scalp defect that results was closed by advancing the posterior scalp flap. Galeal scoring was sometimes necessary to increase the length of the posterior flap.

*Results.*—Twenty-two women (average age 45 years; range 32 to 62 years) presented for correction of their brow position and shape after brow lift surgery. All brows were lowered, and the brow apex was shifted laterally. The medial brow was lowered 3 to 10 mm (average, 6 mm) relative to the intercanthal line. The anterior hairline was lowered 5 to 18 mm (average 12 mm). The repositioning has remained stable over 6 months to 3 years' follow-up. No revisionary surgery has been requested. Two patients had areas of alopecia develop in the posterior scalp flap.

*Conclusions.*—The surgically lifted brow can be lowered and reshaped by advancing, repositioning, and fixing the frontal scalp to the skull.

▶ Most of us feel that many 'brow lifts'[1] give the patient the look of one who just sat on a thumbtack. Some patients like this; however, for those who do not, the authors offer a solution. The thumbtack look can be avoided by knowing the normal brow measurements.

**P. W. McKinney, MD, CM**

*Reference*

1. McKinney P, Raymond DM, Mark LZ. Criteria for the forehead lift. *Aesthetic Plast Surg.* 1991;15:141-147.

---

**Attractiveness of Eyebrow Position and Shape in Females Depends on the Age of the Beholder**
Feser DK, Gründl M, Eisenmann-Klein M, et al (Univ of Regensburg, Germany)
*Aesthetic Plast Surg* 31:154-160, 2007

---

*Background.*—Great diversity exists among individuals with respect to eyebrow position and shape, and the notion of an "ideal" eyebrow has changed quite significantly over the past several decades.

*Methods.*—This study compared three different variations of eyebrows. One variation was the arched eyebrow with the maximum height in the middle. The other two variations had their maximum height in the lateral third, but differed in their position (high vs low). For each of the seven female portraits presented, three variations were generated using morphing software. A total of 357 subjects, 12 to 85 years of age, compared these variations and ranked each woman individually, with respect to perceived attractiveness.

*Results.*—The data show that the preference for a specific eyebrow shape depends on a person's age. Young subjects up to 30 years of age preferred eyebrows in a lower position, and ruled out arched eyebrows. Subjects older than 50 years stated exactly the opposite preference.

*Conclusion.*—First, there is not one single beauty ideal for eyebrows, but at least three. The ideal a person prefers depends on his or her age. Second, because trends are generally introduced by young people and not by older individuals, and the young tend to prefer eyebrows in a lower position, it seems plausible to assume that the trend currently appears to be moving away from arched eyebrows toward lower positioned eyebrows with a maximum height in the lateral third.

▶ This article emphasizes the culture, ethnic, and now age-related concepts of beauty. How often do we see the surgeon's imprint rather than, perhaps, the patient's? Forehead lift is a perfect example, as many of us feel that the postoperative results we see are too high, and the patient looks surprised (in spite of their age). It is best to ask the patients to demonstrate what their concept of brow position is.

**P. W. McKinney, MD, CM**

---

## The Influence of Brow Shape on the Perception of Facial Form and Brow Aesthetics

Baker SB, Dayan JH, Crane A, et al (Georgetown Univ Hosp, Washington, DC)
*Plast Reconstr Surg* 119:2240-2247, 2007

---

*Background.*—Previous studies have described the ideal shape of the aesthetic brow. These studies were based on fashion models, who typically have ideal oval faces. In people with different facial shapes, makeup artists modify brow shape to give the illusion of an oval shape. The purpose of this investigation was to compare the classically described ideal brow to the modified brow for each facial shape.

*Methods.*—The faces of five models were morphed into round, square, oval, and long facial shapes. The eyebrows were digitally removed. A makeup artist drew the brows specifically for each facial shape. In a second set of prints, the brow shape was based on the previously published criteria. Seventy-eight people were asked which face they believed was more aesthetic.

*Results.*—There was no significant difference between the classic and the modified eyebrow in the oval or round facial shapes. In the square and long facial shapes, the modified brow was found to be more attractive in 62.7 percent and 58.7 percent of the subjects, which is statistically significant ($p < 0.05$).

*Conclusions.*—The ideal brow may differ from the classic description when applied to the long or square face. In long faces, a flatter brow may give the illusion of fullness. In the square face, an accentuated lateral curvature may help soften the angles of the face. It may be difficult to achieve these modifications surgically, but it is important to be aware of the effect that brow shape has on facial shape.

▶ Permanently shaping the brows, surgically, without direct scars, which are noticeable, is problematical. They can be raised on block and put more emphasis, placed either medially or laterally, with endoscopic or open scalp techniques, but the subtle shapes, obtained with direct incisions, are rarely obtainable. The makeup artist shows us the way to soften facial shapes, but we are not there yet, surgically.

**P. W. McKinney, MD, CM**

---

### Follicular Anatomy of the Anterior Temporal Hairline and Implications for Rhytidectomy

Mowlavi A, Majzoub RK, Cooney DS, et al (private practice, Laguna Beach, CA; Case Western Reserve Univ, Cleveland, OH; Southern Illinois Univ, Springfield)
*Plast Reconstr Surg* 119:1891-1895, 2007

---

*Background.*—Incisions made perpendicular to the hair follicles during anterior frontal hairline brow lifts or forehead shortening procedures, help produce an inconspicuous forehead scar. The success of this "hidden" incision relies on the anteriorly directed frontal hairline follicles and their growth vector. The authors hypothesized that a similar incision could be made perpendicular to the hair follicles in the temple region during rhytidectomy. A well-designed anterior hairline beveled incision over the temple would allow for improved leverage during soft-tissue repositioning and a concealed hairline incision in the temple region.

*Methods.*—Anterior temporal hairline strips 4 cm in length at the level of the lateral canthus were excised from 16 fresh cadavers. Hairline follicles ($n = 227$) were assessed for direction and angle of growth after appropriate tissue preparation and staining (hematoxylin and eosin). The hair follicle angle was analyzed, microscopically, as it approached the epidermis.

*Results.*—The anterior temporal hairline follicles were oriented at a mean angle with the epidermis of 16 ± 3 degrees anteriorly and inferiorly.

*Conclusions.*—The anterior temporal hairline follicles of the scalp are oriented anteriorly and inferiorly with the epidermis, providing the surgical rationale for using a beveled hairline incision angled 30 to 45 degrees to the external skin surface to undercut the distal flap. This incision is perpendicular to, and transects, the temporal hair follicles during rhytidectomy, permitting hair growth through and anterior to the scar. This modified anterior temporal hairline incision reduces visibility of the scar at the hairline for patients in whom scar show and hairstyle versatility are important concerns.

▶ For over a decade, Camirand[1] has made us rethink our concept of hairline incisions always being parallel to the shafts. The Camirand technique goes perpendicular to the shafts, rather than parallel, causing the regrowth through the scar, which affords camouflage.

**P. W. McKinney, MD, CM**

*Reference*

1. Camirand A, Doucet J. A comparison between parallel hairline incisions and perpendicular incisions when performing a face lift. *Plast Reconstr Surg.* 1997; 99:10-15.

---

### Limited Incision Nonendoscopic Brow Lift
Tabatabai N, Spinelli HM (Weill Med College of Cornell Univ, New York)
*Plast Reconstr Surg* 119:1563-1570, 2007

---

*Background.*—The authors compared the nonendoscopic brow lift technique to the popular endoscopic procedure to determine whether it offers a less complex and less expensive, but equally effective, alternative.

*Methods.*—A retrospective comparison of the senior author's experience with the endoscopic brow lift (100 patients; years 1999 to 2004) and the nonendoscopic brow lift (93 patients; years 2002 to 2005) was conducted. Using a three-incision approach for both procedures (one midline and two temporal), endoscopic visualization was used to assist in the last 2 cm of subperiosteal dissection over the superior orbital rim only in the endoscopic technique. In the nonendoscopic technique, this final dissection was performed without the endoscope, and the expected path of the supraorbital and supratrochlear neurovascular bundles, through preoperative marking of their meridians, was respected. Effective brow elevation, operative times, size of incisions, complications, and overall patient satisfaction were compared between groups.

*Results.*—The authors found no significant difference in average brow elevation between the two brow lift groups (4 mm). However, the nonendoscopic brow lift was completed, on average, 20 minutes faster than the endoscopic brow lift (30 minutes versus 50 minutes) and required a smaller incision than the endoscopic brow lift (2 cm versus 2.5 cm). No nonendoscopic patient experienced permanent complications, but one endoscopic patient developed permanent paresthesias of the forehead, secondary to supraorbital/supratrochlear nerve injury. Overall patient satisfaction was equivalent in both groups.

*Conclusions.*—The limited incision nonendoscopic brow lift is a safe and effective alternative to the endoscopic technique. With thorough anatomical knowledge of this region, it offers equivalent brow elevation, shorter operative times, smaller incisions, similarly low complications rates, and patient satisfaction and eliminates the need for costly, and cumbersome, endoscopic equipment.

▶ This requires an excellent knowledge of the anatomy, which is best obtained by cadaver dissections. The technique will limit most of the effect to the medial and central portions of the brow with less to the latter brow, in that it is a blind procedure.

**P. W. McKinney, MD, CM**

---

**A New Method for the Correction of Small Pixie Earlobe Deformities**
Park C (Korea Univ, Seoul)
*Ann Plast Surg* 59:273-276, 2007

---

A fair number of patients show pixie earlobe deformities in East Asia. Some of them also show small earlobes. They request their earlobes enlarged, in addition to the correction of the pixie earlobe deformities. In this article, I propose a new method for the simultaneous correction of the pixie earlobe and the small earlobe deformities. The pixie earlobe deformities were corrected by an upward lifting of a V-shaped flap. The earlobe expansion was performed using autogenous conchal cartilage and dermafat harvested from the paracoccygeal region. The method provides not only mediolateral expansion of the earlobe but also marginal expansion. Between 2002 and 2005, both ears of 6 patients were corrected using this method. The final esthetic results were gratifying to the patients, as well as to the surgeon.

▶ The author describes an excellent technique for an all-way dimensional size increase, and correction, of the pixie earlobe. Albeit small, it does place a scar on the neck. The pixie component, alone, could be corrected by a short scar rhytidectomy, but the size increase can only be accomplished by adding materials, as the authors describe.

**P. W. McKinney, MD, CM**

# Nose

## A Randomized, Controlled Comparison between Arnica and Steroids in the Management of Postrhinoplasty Ecchymosis and Edema
Totonchi A, Guyuron B (Case Western Reserve Univ, Cleveland, OH)
*Plast Reconstr Surg* 120:271-274, 2007

*Background.*—Both arnica and corticosteroids have been suggested for reducing the postoperative edema and bruising associated with rhinoplasty. This study compared the efficacy of these products following rhinoplasty.

*Methods.*—Forty-eight primary rhinoplasty patients were randomized into three groups: group P received 10 mg of dexamethasone (intravenously) intraoperatively, followed by a 6-day oral tapering dose of methyl-prednisone; group A received arnica three times a day for 4 days; and group C received neither agent and served as the control. Three blinded panelists rated the extent of ecchymosis, the intensity of the ecchymosis, and the severity of the edema.

*Results.*—On postoperative day 2, there were no significant differences in the ratings of extent and intensity of ecchymosis among the groups. There was a significant difference for the edema rating ($p < 0.0001$), with group C demonstrating more swelling, compared with groups A and P. In addition, on postoperative day 8, group P demonstrated a significantly larger extent of ecchymosis ($p < 0.05$) and higher intensity of ecchymosis ($p < 0.01$), compared with groups A and C. There were no differences in the magnitude of edema by postoperative day 8 among the three groups. When the differences between day 2 and day 8 ratings were considered, groups A and C exhibited significantly more resolution of ecchymosis by day 8, compared with group P ($p < 0.05$).

*Conclusions.*—This study suggests that both arnica and corticosteroids may be effective in reducing edema during the early postoperative period. Arnica does not appear to provide any benefit with regard to extent and intensity of ecchymosis. The delay in resolution of ecchymosis, for patients receiving corticosteroids, may outweigh the benefit of reducing edema during the early postoperative period.

▶ Blood pressure and surgical trauma have more to do with bruising and edema than any magic pill. Ice pressure, for a few minutes, immediately after the osteotomy, preoperative workup, and blood pressure control intraoperatively, and in the recovery room, go a long way in preventing ecchymosis. Concerning Arnica, a book called *Secrets of the White Buffalo,*[1] which is a description of North American Indian healing arts, quotes the Lakhota Sioux as saying Arnica is toxic if taken internally and is to be used on unbroken skin. The *P.D.R. for Herbal Medicines*[2] states that Arnica, for internal use, is dangerous because of cardiac muscle palsy and mucous membrane hemorrhage. An overriding consideration, concerning herbals, is that there is no standardization in this industry as to strength from factory to factory and country to country, so the ingestants do not know how much they are taking.

P. W. McKinney, MD, CM

References

1. *Secrets of the Sacred White Buffalo North American Healing by Gary Null.* Paramus, New Jersey: Prentice Hall; 1998:189.
2. *P.D.R. for Herbal Medicines.* Montvale, New Jersey: Medical Economics Company; 1998:663.

### The Pyriform Ligament

Rohrich RJ, Hoxworth RE, Thornton JF, et al (University of Texas Southwestern Medical Ctr, Dallas, TX)
*Plast Reconstr Surg* 121:277-281, 2008

*Background.*—Several ligaments are believed to support the nasal tip. Intraoperative dissection has suggested that a broader ligament may exist along the pyriform rim than has been previously noted. This observation, along with the concept that pyriform rim shape may affect nasal tip projection by ligamentous fixation, led to the present study.

*Methods.*—Ten hemifacial fresh cadaver dissections were performed. Sequential dissection was performed of tissue layers aided by magnification with loupes and an operating microscope. The fascial connection between pyriform rim bone and the upper and lower lateral cartilages and to the alar base was noted. The relationship of upper to lower lateral cartilage, and of the investing fascia to the lower lateral cartilage, was defined.

*Results.*—A dense fascial system was noted in all cadaver dissections arising from the periosteum of the pyriform rim. This ligamentous system inserted onto both the upper and lower lateral cartilages. It encompassed the, previously described, lateral sesamoid complex ligament and the ligament between the upper and lower lateral cartilage. This fascia has a consistent anatomical location and spans the pyriform rim from nasal bone to anterior nasal spine.

*Conclusions.*—A ligament exists between the pyriform rim and lateral cartilages and is broader and more expansive than previously described. It encompasses the, previously described, lateral sesamoid complex and the ligament between the upper and lower lateral cartilages. The consistent anatomical origin of this membrane suggests that the term "pyriform ligament" may be appropriate nomenclature. This ligament may be important in translating anatomical shape—and distortion—of the pyriform rim to the nasal cartilages, and may, therefore, affect tip shape, tip projection, and nasal vault architecture.

▶ A broad based ligament has implications when elevating or advancing the tip, especially in "closed rhinoplasty," as if a complete release is not made caudally, a relapsing force remains. Of course, making "space" for the elevation (ie, ventral caudal septum modification), ventral caudal upper laterals, and cephalic lower laterals (alar cartilages) all assist in this elevation. The pyriform portion of cartilage of the lower lateral is usually thin and may consist of several cartilages, referred to as sesamoids, which may hinge the tip and allow elevation. However, this information presented by the authors may explain the unusual combination of a single cartilage and a "sheet ligament" that does not hinge, therefore requiring a release caudally. In closed rhinoplasty, these patients benefit from an extended bipedicle incision, which would release all of these elements.

**P. W. McKinney, MD, CM**

---

**A Surgical Algorithm Using Open Rhinoplasty for Correction of Traumatic Twisted Nose**
Hsiao Y-C, Kao C-H, Wang H-W, et al (Natl Defense Med Ctr, Taipei, Taiwan, Republic of China; Univ of Washington, Seattle)
*Aesthetic Plast Surg* 31:250-258, 2007

---

In this series, the authors present their experience with correction of the traumatic twisted nose in Asians using open rhinoplasty. A standard surgical algorithm was followed to determine treatment strategies for 92 patients with traumatic twisted nose at the Tri-Service General Hospital in Taiwan between 1 August 2001 and 1 June 2004. A retrospective chart review was performed to collect patient data and surgical details. A follow-up self-evaluation survey, regarding satisfaction with nasal function and aesthetics, was distributed to all the participants. All the patients underwent open rhinoplasties under general anesthesia. The 87 males and 5 females were 15 to 53 years of age (mean, 28 years). Their postoperative periods were uneventful and without complications. Patient self-evaluations were largely positive, reporting improvement in nasal function. The authors propose a simple surgical algorithm using open rhinoplasty for optimal correction of traumatic twisted nose deformities. The algorithm, which is adaptable to a variety of anatomic deformities, guides surgical decision making that yields consistently satisfactory functional and aesthetic results (Figs 1 and 2).

▶ The authors present their approach to the correction of traumatic nasal injuries in Asian patients in a large retrospective series, accumulated over the course of 3 years. Their operative approach uses open rhinoplasty under general anesthesia, and it follows a sequence beginning with the nasal pyramid, moving to the septum, and nasal tip cartilage. Ancillary procedures on the septum, trubinates, and bony structures were common. I agree with the authors' observation that correction of the nasal pyramid is most critical in the repair of the twisted nose, and that the open approach aids this aim. As in the series from the United States, levels of patient satisfaction vary, and dissatisfaction with both aesthetics and function approaches 23% in the latter and 19% in the former. It would be of some interest to accumulate large numbers of patients, through collaborative studies, amongst several centers, to determine if

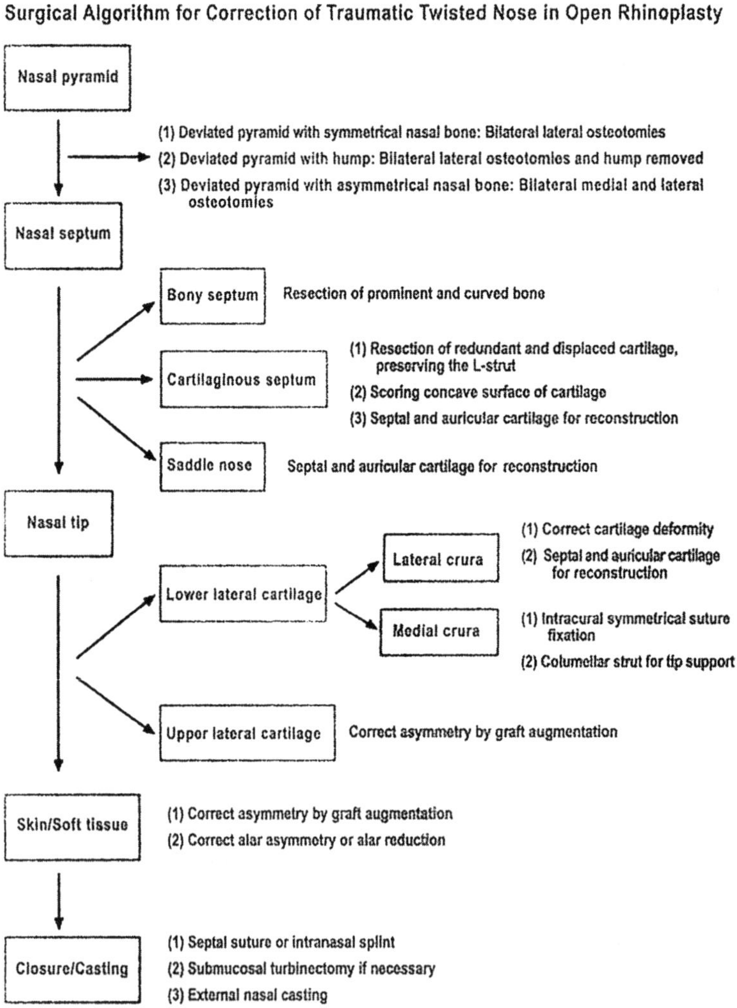

FIGURE 1.—A surgical algorithm for correction of traumatic twisted nose using open rhinoplasty. (Courtesy of Hsiao Y-C, Kao C-H, Wang H-W, et al: A surgical algorithm using open rhinoplasty for correction of traumatic twisted nose. *Aesthetic Plast Surg* 31:250-258, 2007. Reprinted with permission from Springer Science+Business Media, LCC.)

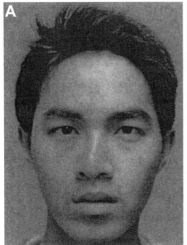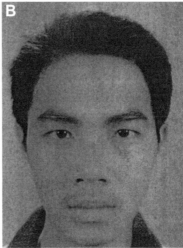

FIGURE 2.—Preoperative (A) and postoperative (B) views of a 23-year-old man with a traumatic twisted nose corrected using open rhinoplasty. (Courtesy of Hsiao Y-C, Kao C-H, Wang H-W, et al: A surgical algorithm using open rhinoplasty for correction of traumatic twisted nose. *Aesthetic Plast Surg* 31:250-258, 2007. Reprinted with permission from Springer Science+Business Media, LCC.)

surgically correctible reasons/or predictions about dissatisfaction factors can be identified to improve postoperative results.

**S. H. Miller, MD, MPH**

## Laminated Dorsal Beam Graft to Eliminate Postoperative Twisting Complications

Swanepoel PF, Fysh R (Nose Clinic, Pretoria, South Africa)
*Arch Facial Plast Surg* 9:285-289, 2007

Preshaped laminated dorsal beam grafts, cut and shaped, from lyophilized rib cartilage eliminate postoperative complications in the correction of saddle depression procedures; lyophilized rib cartilage does not undergo irradiation. Rhinoplasty surgeons traditionally use monounit rib cartilage to correct saddle depressions. During the 3- to 6-month postoperative recovery period, monounit grafts tend to twist and bend, often undermining the shape of the nose. Secondary or revision surgery entails removal of the monounit cartilage. Grafting material used in laminated form is more resilient and flexible than a single unit of similar material. Two-millimeter-thick rib cartilage strips counteract the distorting tendencies of monounit cartilage most effectively. After estimating the dimensions of the required lamination with soft-solid silicone sizers, rib cartilage strips are shaped and sutured into a lamination and then inserted under the skin–soft tissue envelope into the dorsal depression. Surgery is concluded in the normal manner by closing the transcolumella-incision with 6-0 fast absorbing plain cat gut sutures. Results over 3 years (117 dorsal beam procedures from 2003-2005) documented with medical case history follow-ups and postoperative imagery show that the laminations do not bend or revert to the original shape of the rib. Results 4 years after the introduction of the technique suggest that laminations counter the inherent postoperative distortion tendencies of monounit rib cartilage.

▶ Three-year follow-up gives us a decent idea of the durability of this technique, which is designed to prevent warping of monoblock dorsal cartilage grafts. Whether cartilage is the best material is an additional argument, as Peck's iliac bone graft technique offers an abundance of material, it can be harvested under local, and it will never warp. This gets into the whole discussion of bone versus cartilage and autogenous materials versus heterogeneous materials. For further reading on this subject, I suggest an article by Peck et al.[1]

**P. W. McKinney, MD, CM**

*Reference*

1. Peck GC. *Techniques in Aesthetic Rhinoplasty.* New York, London: Gauer Medical Publishing; 1984. Page 140.

---

**Biodegradable polymer membrane used as septal splint**
Watzinger F, Wutzl A, Wanschitz F, et al (Univ Hosp for Craniomaxillofacial and Oral Surgery, Vienna, Austria)
*Int J Oral Maxillofac Surg* 37:473-477, 2008

---

The treatment of a crooked nose is one of the most challenging rhinoplastic procedures. Correction of the abnormally curved or fractured septum has been reported using mostly scoring techniques, septoplasty and submucous resection techniques; cartilaginous spreader grafts can also be sutured to the distorted septum. Extracorporal septal straightening and repositioning/refixation is another useful but difficult technique. A common problem of septal cartilaginous grafting techniques is to harvest enough straight cartilage to correct the deformity. (Other donor sites such as rib cartilage are used, but harvesting additional cartilage is a time-consuming procedure and carries the risk of donor site morbidity.) Recent studies have been published using alloplastic internal splinting of the deformed septum. The use of poly p-dioxanone foils and porous polyethylene has been suggested before. In this study, a novel grafting material, a PolyMax membrane that has potential advantages over both materials, is presented. This is a porous biodegradable polymer made out of 70:30 poly(L-lactide-co-D,L-lactide) that remains stable for at least 7 months. Poly p-dioxanone loses its stability after only 2 months, whereas porous polyethylene is a permeable material that is controversial due to possible complications in cases of membrane exposure and infection. In this

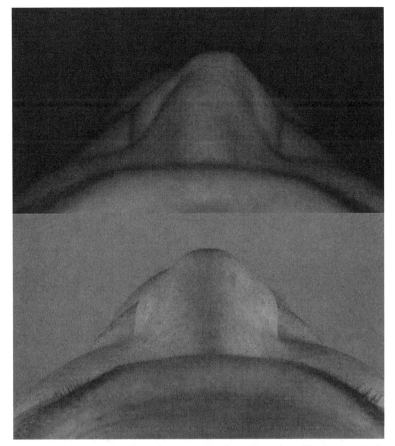

**FIGURE 4.**—Case 2: preoperative and postoperative views of a patient with severely twisted nose. (Reprinted from Watzinger F, Wutzl A, Wanschitz F, et al. Biodegradable polymer membrane used as septal splint. *Int J Oral Maxillofac Surg.* 2008;37:473-477. Copyright 2008, with permission from the International Association of Oral and Maxillofacial Surgeons.)

preliminary report the PolyMax membrane was used successfully in 3 patients (Figs 4-7).

▶ Reliable long-term correction of a crooked nose has, for the most part, been an elusive goal. Procedures to straighten, reconstruct, and fixate the native septal cartilage are difficult, and in many instances fail to maintain the nose in a straightened position. One of the more successful techniques is to harvest other cartilage, usually rib, and form a dorsal strut to "disguise" the deformity. To avoid the need for harvesting cartilage, several authors have proposed using alloplastic materials combined with procedures to straighten and/or reconstruct the native septal cartilage. The authors present their preliminary experience in 3 patients undergoing surgery for a crooked nose with a new biodegradable

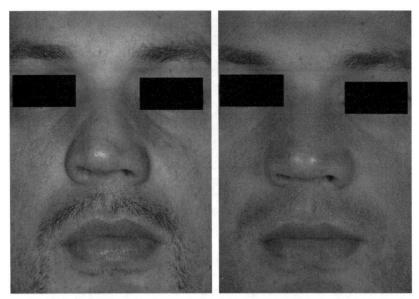

**FIGURE 5.**—Frontal pre- and postoperative views of case 2. (Reprinted from Watzinger F, Wutzl A, Wanschitz F, et al. Biodegradable polymer membrane used as septal splint. *Int J Oral Maxillofac Surg.* 2008;37:473-477. Copyright 2008, with permission from the International Association of Oral and Maxillofacial Surgeons.)

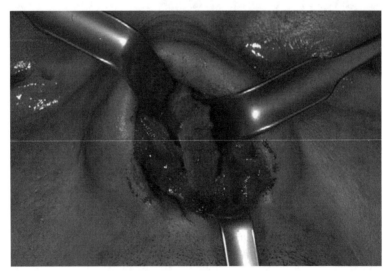

**FIGURE 6.**—Case 2: intraoperative view of septal fracture and deformity. (Reprinted from Watzinger F, Wutzl A, Wanschitz F, et al. Biodegradable polymer membrane used as septal splint. *Int J Oral Maxillofac Surg.* 2008;37:473-477. Copyright 2008, with permission from the International Association of Oral and Maxillofacial Surgeons.)

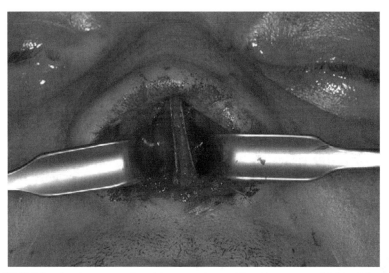

FIGURE 7.—Case 2: reconstruction of the septum interpositioned between two PolyMax foils, fixed with PDS sutures. (Reprinted from Watzinger F, Wutzl A, Wanschitz F, et al. Biodegradable polymer membrane used as septal splint. *Int J Oral Maxillofac Surg.* 2008;37:473-477. Copyright 2008, with permission from the International Association of Oral and Maxillofacial Surgeons.)

alloplastic material, a polymer of 70:30 poly(lactide-co-D,C-lactide) manufactured by Synthes. It is quite flexible and easily modified during the surgical procedure. The material is said to biodegrade in 1-3 years.[1] The results appear to be promising at an average follow-up of 7 months, however, all had airway obstruction due to edema at the early postoperative stages. In 2 patients it resolved, but 1 of the 3 patients still has a degree of airway obstruction after 6 months. Long term results (1-2 years) in a much larger series of patients are obviously necessary.

**S. H. Miller, MD, MPH**

*Reference*

1. Schmidmaier G, Baehr K, Mohr S, et al. Biodegradable polylactide membranes for bone defect coverage: biocompatibility testing, radiological and histological evaluation in a sheep model. *Clin Oral Implants Res.* 2006;17:439-444.

---

**Allogenous Cartilage Graft Versus Autogenous Cartilage Graft in Augmentation Rhinoplasty: A Decade of Clinical Experience**
Tosun Z, Karabekmez FE, Keskin M, et al (Selcuk Univ, Konya, Turkey)
*Aesthet Plast Surg* 32:252-260, 2008

---

Cartilage grafts have great value in augmentation rhinoplasty. For most surgeons, an autogenous cartilage graft is the first choice in rhinoplasty because of its resistance to infection and resorption. On the other hand, an allogenous cartilage graft might be preferred over an autogenous graft to avoid additional morbidity and lengthened operating time. Allogenous cartilage grafts not only have the advantage of averting donor site morbidity but also are resistant to infection, resembling autogenous cartilage grafts. The authors present their experience with 41 patients who underwent augmentation rhinoplasty using 22 autogenous and 19 allogenous cartilage grafts between June 1994 and August 2004. For evaluation of adequate augmentation rates, photographic analyses were performed on preoperative, early postoperative, and late postoperative photographs from all the patients. To assess patient satisfaction, the Facial Appearance Sorting Test (FAST) was applied preoperatively and late postoperatively in both groups. These results were compared, and it was concluded that in terms of resorption, there was no difference in the early and late postoperative follow-up data between allogenous and autogenous cartilage grafts. Evaluation of the preoperative and early postoperative photographic outcomes showed statistically significant differences with respect to adequate augmentation rates between the two groups. The FAST scores showed statistically significant differences between preoperative and late postoperative outcomes. There were no infections in the two groups of patients.

▶ When the septum and/or the ears are insufficient in volume for a cartilage, the authors have demonstrated an alternative technique comparing 19 allogenous grafts of solvent dehydrated human costal cartilage, which show an equal lack of absorption, with 22 autogenous grafts in a follow-up that extended as long as 10 years. This was judged to be statistically significant. If this holds up it means that if cartilage is needed, the autogenous costal cartilage with its potential problematic donor site may not be needed, and indeed a "shelf" product will do as well as autogenous cartilage with regard to infection (none in either group) or reabsorption (the same in both the auto and allo groups). Note that the authors used only closed rhinoplasty for access with its potential therefore of better vascularity by leaving the columellar arteries intact. Although skin conditions (vascularity ± scars) were not mentioned by the authors, the photos of the 7 patients illustrated indicate a soft, pliable vascular skin cover, which is an important indicator for success of any foreign material insertion in the nose. In addition, the reports of absence of HIV in the costal cartilages even in HIV-infected patients makes this an attractive alternative.[1]

**P. W. McKinney, MD, CM**

*Reference*

1. Bujia J, Zietz C, Randolph P, Wilmes E, Gurtler L. Absence of HIV-1 DNA in cartilage from HIV positive patients. *Eur Arch Otorhinolaryngol.* 1994;251: 347-349.

### Management of severe tip ptosis in closed rhinoplasty: the horizontal columellar strut

Margulis A, Harel M (Hadassah Med Ctr of Hebrew Univ, Jerusalem; private practice, Tel Aviv, Israel)
*J Plast Reconstr Aesthetic Surg* 60:400-406, 2007

*Background.*—Tip ptosis is a relatively common nasal deformity, with an incidence as high as 72% in rhinoplasty patients. Different techniques were described for surgical correction of the droopy tip, such as the lateral crural steel, the lateral crural overlay, the tongue-in-groove technique and others. Most authors agreed that an external rhinoplasty approach is necessary for effectively conducting the alar cartilage-modifying techniques mentioned above.

*Methods.*—In this article, we challenge this paradigm and introduce an efficient method for aesthetic correction of severe tip ptosis through an internal rhinoplasty approach. Twenty-three patients with severe ptosis of the nasal tip were operated on by the senior author (MH), between 2000 and 2005, using the described technique. After carrying out the necessary manœuvres to achieve the desired tip rotation (reduction of cephalic border of alar cartilages, modification of the caudal septum, reduction of upper lateral cartilages), the desired tip position was maintained with the horizontal columellar strut, whose initial operative description appears here.

*Results.*—The desired rotation and projection were maintained in all but three patients over the first year after the surgery. In three patients, we observed some loss of tip projection after 1 year. We did not witness complications directly related to the horizontal columellar strut.

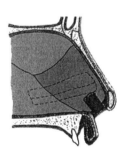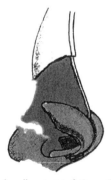

FIGURE 1.—Schematic diagram of the horizontal columellar strut technique. (Left) The cephalic portion of the strut is affixed to the caudal cartilaginous septum with clear nylon sutures at the level of the midportion of the medial crura. (Right) The caudal edge of the strut is allowed to lie freely in between the medial crura, in a way that resembles tongue-in-groove. (Courtesy of Margulis A, Harel M. Management of severe tip ptosis in closed rhinoplasty: the horizontal columellar strut. *J Plast Reconstr Aesthetic Surg.* 2007;60:400-406, with permission from British Association of Plastic, Reconstructive and Aesthetic Surgeons.)

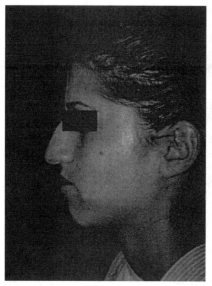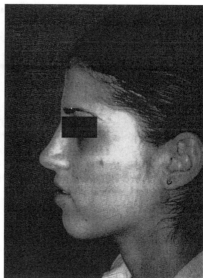

FIGURE 3.—(Left) Preoperative views of a patient with a broad, droopy nasal tip with an adequate amount of projection. (Right) Postoperative views of the same patient 1.2 years after the operation using the horizontal columellar strut technique, showing increase in nasal tip projection, rotation and definition. Additional manœuvres included cephalic trim of the alar cartilages, conservative lowering of the nasal dorsum and lateral osteotomies. (Courtesy of Margulis A, Harel M. Management of severe tip ptosis in closed rhinoplasty: the horizontal columellar strut. *J Plast Reconstr Aesthetic Surg.* 2007;60:400-406, with permission from British Association of Plastic, Reconstructive and Aesthetic Surgeons.)

*Conclusion.*—The horizontal columellar strut is an efficient tool for stabilising the corrected position of a severely ptotic nasal tip. We recommend adding the horizontal columellar strut to the array of available rhinoplasty techniques (Figs 1 and 3).

▶ This horizontal graft, in the area of the nasal spine/columella, will offer the illusion of elevation by lowering the columella nasal spine appearance. The use of this depends on the preoperative appearance, as the patient with a hypertrophic spine may not be a good candidate for this procedure. Note how much graft is required in this area to effect a small change.

**P. W. McKinney, MD, CM**

---

### Effect of Nasal Tip Surgery on Asian Noses Using the Transdomal Suture Technique

Jang T-Y, Choi Y-S, Jung Y-G, et al (Inha Univ, Incheon, Korea)
*Aesthetic Plast Surg* 31:174-178, 2007

---

The past two decades have ushered in a new era of nasal tip surgery. The new philosophy focuses on preserving and reorienting nasal tip structures.

Modern suture techniques can give predictable results because of more precise suture placement. Only a few reports, however, have objectively evaluated the suture techniques for Asians. Accordingly, the authors aimed to assess the efficacy of the tip suture technique through projection and rotation analysis. We focused on transdomal sutures because they involve one of the most popular suture techniques. Preoperative and postoperative photographs of 85 patients who underwent rhinoplasty at Inha University Hospital, between June 2002 and June 2004, were analyzed. The patients were categorized into four groups according to the techniques used. Tip projection was measured by the modified Heuzinger's method and tip rotation by the nasolabial angle. The pre- and postoperative indexes were compared within each group and among the four groups. Paired and unpaired $t$ tests were used for statistical analysis. When the pre- and postoperative indexes were compared within each group, only the combined technique (transdomal suture with onlay graft) showed significant tip projection improvement. All tip surgeries resulted in insignificant tip rotation increase. Comparison among the four groups showed no significant difference based on the type of tip surgery performed. The suture technique has many advantages, although it has some limitations with Asian noses, especially, if used alone. Therefore, we recommend using the suture technique in combination with other tip surgical procedures, such as onlay grafts, to achieve significant tip projection.

▶ This analysis applies to all "thin alar cartilages" and not just Asian ones. The use of tip grafts requires strong lateral and medial support. Otherwise, the pressure of the grafting may cause the projection to "melt" into the face.

**P. W. McKinney, MD, CM**

---

**Septocolumellar Suture in Closed Rhinoplasty**
Tezel E, Numanoğlu A (Marmara Univ, Istanbul, Turkey)
*Ann Plast Surg* 59:268-272, 2007

---

Several surgeons advise a variety of tip sutures and describe their own techniques in open approach. Septocolumellar suture is one of them, and it can be described as a loop suture between the medial crura and caudal septum. Although some of the articles mention that it can be applied in closed rhinoplasty, there is no description of the technical details. This paper presents indications, technical steps, and advantages of the septocolumellar suture in closed rhinoplasty.

After completing the classic sequence of the endonasal extramucous technique, the medial crural cartilages are dissected from the overlying skin at the midcolumellar level, keeping the distal fibrous attachments between the anterior columellar skin and these cartilages intact. A 5/0 or 4/0 Prolene (Ethicon Ltd, UK) with a round needle is passed, penetrating both the medial crura and then the caudal septum. Depending on the penetration level of this suture, the tip projection can be increased or decreased, the tip can be rotated, and columellar show can be corrected. This suture also makes the medial crura of the alar cartilages and septum rigidly fixed together, thus providing stability. Depending on the experience gained in 433 primary and 62 secondary rhinoplasty cases since 2000, it can be claimed that this technique, presenting an alternative to the open approach in many cases and expanding the borders of closed approach, allows one to manipulate the tip and columella easily with closed rhinoplasty and provides a significant decrease in the suboptimal results and number of complications.

▶ Aufricht[1] called this suture his "orthopedic stitch," which he used as a last step in closure of his rhinoplasties to "set" the nasal tip in the manner the author describes. He used a 3-0 silk external suture for this purpose. Note the author's prediction of more closed rhinoplasties, as opposed to the current phase of opens; and if I may add one myself, we will be doing more rhinoplasties in the seated position.

**P. W. McKinney, MD, CM**

*Reference*

1. Gustov Aufricht, personal communication to Dr. Peter McKinney.

## A Simplified Use of Septal Extension Graft to Control Nasal Tip Location
Seyhan A, Ozden S, Ozaslan U, et al (Celal Bayar Univ, Manisa, Turkey)
*Aesthetic Plast Surg* 31:506-511, 2007

*Background.*—For defining the shape and projection of the nasal tip, the bilateral and symmetric batten-type septal extension grafts proposed by Byrd and colleagues have drawbacks. The main problems are stiffness of the nasal tip and thickening of the septum in the nasal valve area.

*Methods.*—Since 1998, unilateral single-batten grafts, and more frequently, bilateral asymmetric batten grafts as compared with Byrd's bilateral symmetric application, have been used for 72 patients in our facility.

*Results.*—At the 6-month postoperative follow-up assessment, tip projection was found to be satisfactory in 61 patients. Less than desired projection occurred in three cases and overprojection in two cases. Nasal lobule deviation was evident in one patient. The loss of the columellar break point was evident in five cases.

*Conclusion.*—Unilateral or asymmetric bilateral batten grafts facilitate adjustment of the nasal tip intraoperatively. This technique results in a more pliable nasal tip in the horizontal plane. Construction of a three-layered cartilage in the nasal valve area is not needed, and the nasal airway is preserved. With this modification, a reliable and predictable nasal tip location is obtained with a minimum of graft usage.

▶ The question is gaining enough experience as to when an open rhinoplasty and batten grafts are necessary. A thin skin envelope and amorphous structures are always candidates, but what if the milder problems can be handled with simpler techniques?

**P. W. McKinney, MD, CM**

**Hockey-Stick Vertical Dome Division Technique for Overprojected and Broad Nasal Tips**
Chang CWD, Simons RL (Univ of Missouri, Columbia; Univ of Miami, FL; MIAMI Institute for Age Management and Intervention, Miami)
*Arch Facial Plast Surg* 10:88-92, 2008

*Objectives.*—To discuss overprojected and broad nasal tips, to overview treatment options, and to relate our experience with the hockey-stick technique.

*Design.*—A retrospective review (1975-2005) was conducted. Patients were selected from a computerized rhinoplasty database of operative cases. The database was used to extract a subset population that had received the hockey-stick tip procedure and had follow-up data for 1 year or more after surgery. Medical records and photographs were also analyzed in this review of results and complications.

*Results.*—The hockey-stick modification of vertical dome division was used in 137 patients (9.9% of the rhinoplasties in the computerized database). Of these, 64 patients had 1 year or more of follow-up. Complications referable to the nasal tip (eg, bossae, persistent tip projection, and alar asymmetry) were seen in 8 patients (13%). Revisions for tip-related problems were performed in 4 patients (6%).

*Conclusions.*—The hockey-stick technique is an effective method for nasal tip deprojection and narrowing via an endonasal approach. The length of follow-up in this patient population allows good long-term evaluation of this technique.

▶ The dome division techniques were originally used to project narrow and simultaneously raise the nasal tip. Modifications, such as the "hockey-stick," deproject and narrow the tip. The critics of dome division techniques point to the development of sharp edges and inspiratory collapse, especially in thin-skinned individuals. I find dome division useful in some individuals, especially snubbed, plunging, wide tips, but I do reserve it for thick skin. If this technique is indicated in thin-skin patients, the addition of a cartilage cap over the potentially sharp edges of the medial crura may hide future problems, and at times a fascia graft as well. It is a useful technique in experienced hands. The senior author of this article is known for his skills in applying dome division techniques.

P. W. Mckinney, MD, CM

## The Spreader Flap in Primary Rhinoplasty
Gruber RP, Park E, Newman J, et al (Stanford Univ, CA; Univ of California, San Francisco; private practice, Campbell, CA; et al)
*Plast Reconstr Surg* 119:1903-1910, 2007

*Background.*—In a primary rhinoplasty that requires a humpectomy, the dorsal aspect of the upper lateral cartilages is commonly discarded. Many of these patients need spreader grafts to reconstruct the middle third of the nose. However, it is possible to reconstruct the upper lateral cartilages into "spreader flaps" that act much like spreader grafts.

*Methods.*—A tunnel is created on the underside of the upper lateral cartilage, which is released from the cartilaginous septum and also from its attachment to the nasal bone (medially). It is then rolled on itself to make a spreader flap, which is secured with sutures. Scoring along the dorsal edge of the upper lateral cartilage may be necessary. The flap is then secured to the dorsal edge of the reduced dorsal septum.

*Results.*—In 21 patients who underwent an open approach (and four patients who underwent the closed approach), the spreader flap almost always reconstructed the middle third of the nose. It was easy to execute in the open approach but difficult in the closed approach. At surgery, two patients undergoing the open approach and one patient undergoing the closed approach needed spreader grafts because the flaps were too narrow. Postoperatively, only one patient (operated on by the open approach) exhibited inadequate nasal width.

*Conclusions.*—Spreader grafts are the standard for reconstructing the middle third of the nose; however, the spreader flap avoids harvesting and carving cartilage for those grafts. In the open approach, the technique is easy to execute. Conclusions could not be drawn regarding the long-term success with the closed approach.

▶ Although the authors, with their skills, may be able to do this closed, it is exceedingly difficult, and a free graft, placed close to the apex of the vault on the septal side, is an accurate and relatively straightforward procedure even in closed cases. This pocket is made by hydrodissection of the nasal septal lining, first followed by a sharp Joseph elevator to make the pocket just dorsal to the apex. This minimizes the risk of tears.

P. W. Mckinney, MD, CM

### Reducing the Incidence of Revision Rhinoplasty

Thomson C, Mendelsohn M (St George's Med Ctr, Christchurch, New Zealand; Sydney Ear Nose and Throat and Facial Cosmetic Day Surgery, NSW, Australia)
*J Otolaryngol* 36:130-134, 2007

*Objectives.*—To evaluate reasons for revision rhinoplasty in a tertiary care setting to help reduce the incidence of revision rhinoplasty.

*Methods.*—Retrospective review of 184 consecutive revision rhinoplasty cases performed by a single surgeon, evaluating the major reasons for patients seeking revision rhinoplasty surgery.

*Results.*—The senior author performed 539 rhinoplasty cases during the period January 2001 to June 2003. 184 were revision cases. Within this group, 56 were the author's own revisions, and 128 had undergone primary surgery by "other surgeons." Major revision indications were airway in 109, crookedness in 70, residual hump in 31 and irregularity in 25 cases. Less common problems included inadequate reduction, tip asymmetry, tip bossae, saddle deformity and change of mind. The incidence of airway restriction and crookedness in the author group was significantly less than in the other surgeon group ($p < .0001$ and $p = .0002$, respectively). Other indications did not differ significantly between the groups.

*Conclusion.*—The pattern of problems requiring revision rhinoplasty is changing as the improved skills of the surgeon are countered by the increased demands of the patient. The high incidence of nasal obstruction following rhinoplasty reminds us that attention to the airway should not be compromised in the focus on cosmetic outcome. Crookedness of the nose has become a notable complaint by a discriminating public. All patients undergoing primary rhinoplasty need advice that revision

TABLE 1.—Indications for Revision Rhinoplasty by Group

| Indication | All Cases ($N = 184$), $n$ (%) | Author Group ($n = 56$), $n$ (%) | Other Surgeons Group ($n = 128$), $n$ (%) | $p$ Value (Fisher Exact Test) |
|---|---|---|---|---|
| Airway | 109 (59) | 14 (25) | 95 (74) | <.0001 |
| Crooked | 70 (38) | 10 (18) | 60 (47) | .0002 |
| Airway and crooked | 42 (23) | 0 (0) | 42 (33) | <.0001 |
| Hump | 31 (17) | 13 (23) | 18 (14) | .1382 |
| Irregularity | 25 (14) | 9 (16) | 16 (13) | .4942 |
| Too big | 24 (13) | 6 (11) | 18 (14) | .6387 |
| Pollybeak | 9 (5) | 0 (0) | 9 (7) | .0590 |
| Tip bossae | 9 (5) | 3 (5) | 6 (5) | 1.0000 |
| Tip asymmetry | 12 (7) | 1 (2) | 11 (9) | .1098 |
| Saddle | 7 (4) | 0 (0) | 7 (6) | .1030 |

(Courtesy of Thomson C, Mendelsohn M. Reducing the incidence of revision rhinoplasty. *J Otolaryngol.* 2007; 36:130-134.)

rhinoplasty may be necessary either during or after the healing phase (Table 1).

▶ Changes in education are going to focus on different areas from generation to generation. For example, a low dorsum is less common today, as we emphasize an elegant natural line; but do not assume that all patients want this, and the simulation images can be of help here. The common complaints a patient brings are: a ball remaining on the tip, breathing problems, crooked nose, and spicules (either bone or cartilage). Occasionally, complaints are of a residual hump, and we, as surgeons, notice the inverted V deformity on the dorsum now that we have camouflage and spreader techniques.

**P. W. McKinney, MD, CM**

# Trunk, Genitalia, and Extremities

## Noninvasive Body Contouring by Focused Ultrasound: Safety and Efficacy of the Contour I Device in a Multicenter, Controlled, Clinical Study

Teitelbaum SA, Burns JL, Kubota J, et al (Univ of California, Santa Monica; Dallas Plastic Surgery Inst; Tokyo Med Univ; et al)
*Plast Reconstr Surg* 120:779-789, 2007

*Background.*—The removal of unwanted body fat using a noninvasive technique is desirable to patients and physicians. The authors describe a controlled, multicenter, clinical trial assessing the safety and efficacy of a focused therapeutic ultrasound device for noninvasive body contouring.

*Methods.*—Eligible healthy adult subjects were enrolled to the experimental group, or the control group, at five sites. The experimental group received one treatment with the Contour I device (UltraShape Ltd., Tel Aviv, Israel) in the abdomen, thighs, or flanks, and were evaluated over a 12-week period. Efficacy outcomes were reduction of circumference and fat thickness. Circumference reduction was compared with the untreated group and with an untreated area (thigh) within the treated group. Safety monitoring included laboratory testing (including serum lipids), pulse oximetry, and liver ultrasound.

*Results.*—One hundred sixty-four subjects participated in the study (137 subjects in the experimental group and 27 in the control, untreated group). A single Contour I treatment was safe and well tolerated and produced a mean reduction of approximately 2 cm in treatment area circumference and approximately 2.9 mm in skin fat thickness. The majority of the effect was achieved within 2 weeks and was sustained at 12 weeks. No clinically significant changes in the measured safety parameters were recorded. Seven adverse events were reported, all of which were anticipated, mild, and resolved within the study period.

*Conclusion.*—The Contour I device provides a safe and effective noninvasive technology for body contouring.

▶ Are these modalities worthy? The study lacks control, uses the inaccurate pinch test as the end point, and is funded by the manufacturer. Yet, the photographs demonstrate modest reductions at 12 weeks. If permanent, where does the fat go? Why is there no induration? We always hope that one of these noninvasive techniques actually proves itself.

**P. W. McKinney, MD, CM**

---

**Progressive Tension Sutures in the Prevention of Postabdominoplasty Seroma: A Prospective, Randomized, Double-Blind Clinical Trial**
Andrades P, Prado A, Danilla S, et al (Univ of Chile, Santiago)
*Plast Reconstr Surg* 120:935-946, 2007

---

*Background.*—The purpose of this study was to evaluate the seroma reduction capabilities of progressive tension sutures and compare them with the conventional use of drains.

*Methods.*—Sixty female patients were randomized into four groups: group 1 (control, no drains, and no progressive tension sutures), group 2 (progressive tension sutures alone), group 3 (drains alone), and group 4 (progressive tension sutures and drains). All patients underwent a classic abdominoplasty and drains were left for 7 days in the corresponding groups. Clinical and ultrasound assessments were performed 2 weeks after the operation by blinded evaluators. Punctures, volumes, nonseroma complications, and aesthetic outcome were also measured.

*Results.*—Surgical time was 50 minutes longer in groups 2 and 4. Drain outputs were higher in group 3 than in group 4. The clinical and ultrasound seroma frequency was 35 percent and 90 percent respectively, without significant differences among the groups. The control group was interrupted at 10 patients because of considerably larger seromas and an increased amount of punctures needed for treatment. No differences were found in the other groups. There were no differences with respect to complication rates and aesthetic outcome after follow-up.

*Conclusions.*—Progressive tension sutures increase surgical time, reduce drain outputs, and have the same clinical and ultrasound seroma frequency as the use of drains alone. The combination of both methods simultaneously does not add any advantages. However, complications and interventions increase if at least one of them is not used. The mechanism of action of progressive tension sutures could be the compartmentalization of the fluid collection under the flap facilitating absorption.

▶ "To drain or not to drain" is the question in all of our surgeries, and this always stimulates debate. For a facelift, unless it is wet (leaking like herbal or aspirin ingestions), I do not drain but rather use a loose subcutaneous closure, which allows fluid to escape. For abdominoplasty, I use suction drains for 5 to 7 days because of the relatively large undermined area in relation to the skin incision and the mobility of the muscles.

**P. W. McKinney, MD, CM**

**The Maltese cross technique: umbilical reconstruction after dermolipectomy**
Rogliani M, Silvi E, Arpino A, et al (Univ "Tor Vergata" Rome)
*J Plast Reconstr Aesthetic Surg* 60:1036-1038, 2007

A simple and easy technique for reconstruction of the umbilicus was devised, with emphasis on forming walls of the umbilicus and a depression in a caudal direction. A quite satisfactory result was obtained. A permanent and sufficient depression for the umbilicus can be expected as a result

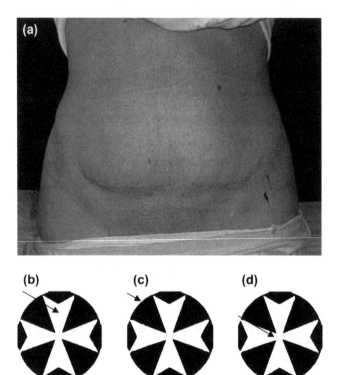

FIGURE 1.—a. Pre-operative situation. b. Maltese cross design: White areas represent the flap without epithelium. c. Maltese cross design: Black zone represent the areas with epithelium. d. Maltese cross design: Sutura point on wraps of the rectum of the abdomen. (Reprinted from Rogliani M, Silvi E, Arpino A, et al. The Maltese cross technique: umbilical reconstruction after dermolipectomy. *J Plast Reconstr Aesthetic Surg.* 2007;60:1036-1038. Copyright 2007, with permission from the British Association of Plastic, Reconstructive and Aesthetic Surgeons.)

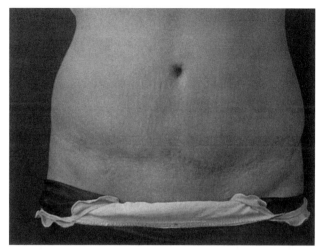

FIGURE 5.—Post operative. (Reprinted from Rogliani M, Silvi E, Arpino A, et al. The Maltese cross technique: umbilical reconstruction after dermolipectomy. *J Plast Reconstr Aesthetic Surg.* 2007;60:1036-1038. Copyright 2007, with permission from the British Association of Plastic, Reconstructive and Aesthetic Surgeons.)

of three-dimensional formation of walls. We also obtained a natural-looking neo-umbilicus (Figs 1 and 5).

▶ A nice result that fulfills the criteria of no circular scar, but it is also very complex. Alternatives may be the curved H incision or even simpler if a concurrent abdominoplasty being done is the defatting with a tack down of the dermis to the rectus fascia, creating a reasonable umbilicus.

**P. W. McKinney, MD, CM**

---

**Increased Intraabdominal Pressure in Abdominoplasty: Delineation of Risk Factors**

Huang GJ, Bajaj AK, Gupta S, et al (Loma Linda Univ, CA; Univ of Cincinnati, OH)

*Plast Reconstr Surg* 119:1319-1325, 2007

---

*Background.*—Abdominoplasty is associated with a 1.1 percent risk of deep venous thrombosis. This has been attributed to rectus plication causing intraabdominal hypertension, known to effect decreased venous return, venous stasis, and thus thrombosis. The authors conducted a pilot study to determine which components of the abdominoplasty procedure (i.e., general anesthesia, flexion of the bed, plication, and/or binder placement) may elevate intraabdominal pressures and whether this was clinically relevant.

*Methods.*—Twelve abdominoplasty and 10 breast reduction (control) patients were enrolled, prospectively. Intraabdominal pressure was transduced through the bladder before plication in the supine and flexed positions, after plication in both positions, after skin closure in the flexed position, and on postoperative day 1, with and without a binder in the flexed position.

*Results.*—All intraabdominal pressures measured were clinically insignificant (<20 mm Hg). A statistically significant increase was found from flexion of the bed (mean difference, $3.80 \pm 2.0$, $p < 0.001$, in the control group; and $4.39 \pm 1.68$, $p < 0.001$, in the study group); rectus plication (mean difference, $2.78 \pm 2.11$, $p = 0.001$, in the supine position; and $2.03 \pm 2.48$, $p = 0.016$, in the flexed position); and binder placement ($2.63$ mm Hg for no binder versus $4.5$ mm Hg with binder, $p = 0.004$). Both groups also showed an increase from preoperative to skin closure (mean difference, $2.03 \pm 6.7$, $p = 0.035$, for the control group; and $2.83 \pm 3.97$, $p = 0.031$, for the study group), suggesting general anesthesia as a risk factor.

*Conclusions.*—This study confirms the effect of rectus plication on increasing intraabdominal pressures but also implicates bed position, binder placement, and general anesthetic as risk factors. A larger study is needed to clarify the role of these variables in elevating intraabdominal pressure during abdominoplasty.

▶ Preoperative condition is important, as well. Intraoperatively, each step in the procedure that the authors demonstrate leads to increased pressure and, therefore, increased risk of embolism. Rectus plication, binders, bed position, and general anesthesia all increase the pressure. We can control binders and beds. We can reduce the time of anesthesia and prepare our patients, preoperatively, with physical therapy.

**P. W. McKinney, MD, CM**

---

**Antibiotic use in abdominoplasty: prospective analysis of 207 cases**
Sevin A, Senen D, Sevin K, et al (Ankara Numune Training and Research Hosp, Turkey; Ankara Univ, Turkey)
*J Plast Reconstr Aesthetic Surg* 60:379-382, 2007

---

The increasing demand for plastic surgery of the abdomen has also increased the number of complications, some of them very difficult to manage. It has been stated that antibiotics are unquestionably effective in preventing postoperative wound infections. In the present study, we aimed to provide guidelines for the use of prophylactic antibiotics in abdominoplasty operations. A prospective study was planned on 207 patients. Three study groups were formed, according to the administration of antibiotics, as follows: group 1, no antibiotics; group 2, preoperative antibiotics only; and group 3, both preoperative and postoperative antibiotics. Twenty patients showed bacterial growth in the intraoperative bacterial culture. There was significant difference in the incidence of infection between groups 1 and 2, groups 1 and 3, but there was no difference between groups 2 and 3. In conclusion, we recommend a single preoperative dose of intravenous antibiotic to prevent infection and also secure the patient from antibiotic side effects.

▶ This seems to be an effective strategy. The use of antibiotics in clean cases requires very large numbers to study adequately, so we do not often have good data in these situations. When antibiotics are used, they should be intravenous, just before surgery, so that the blood level is elevated when the wound is open. In clean/contaminated (for instance intraoral) cases, the indications for usage are clearer. In clean cases with prostheses, it is still very debatable.

**P. W. McKinney, MD, CM**

---

**Pyoderma gangrenosum following abdominoplasty—a rare complication**
Patel AJK, O'Broin ES (Leicester Royal Infirmary, England; Cork Univ Hosp, Ireland)
*Eur J Plast Surg* 29:317-319, 2007

---

*Background.*—Pyoderma gangrenosum is characterized by progressive noninfective skin ulcerations. Pathergy is the term when this occurs at the site of surgery. Nonsurgical treatment is generally recommended for this rare condition. A case occurring after abdominoplasty was described.

*Case Report.*—Woman, 41, had a scar from a Lanz incision as well as scars located at the infraumbilical midline and lower abdomen (Pfannensteil incisions). She underwent a standard abdominoplasty and had an uneventful immediate postoperative course. She had continued to smoke cigarettes against medical advice during the perioperative period. At routine follow-up 1 week after surgery, her wounds were healing nicely. Wound breakdown of the right end of the transverse scar and umbilical wounds prompted her return 3 weeks after surgery; the condition progressed over the following 2 days. Necrotizing fasciitis could not be ruled out. Intravenous antibiotics were begun, and she underwent minimal debridement. Close inspection showed the wounds had violet borders with pus in the dermis, suggestive of pyoderma gangrenosum. No organisms were detected on Gram staining, but histologic analysis of tissue samples yielded findings consistent with pyodrema gangrenosum. Cyclosporin was begun after consultation with the dermatology team concurred with the presumptive diagnosis. The wounds responded to the medication plus regular dressings. After 3 weeks split-thickness skin grafts were used to repair the wounds, followed by another course of cyclosporin. No further complications developed.

*Conclusions.*—Pyoderma gangrenosum occurs in four variants (ulcerative, pustular, bullous, and vegetative), and the patient described had the characteristics of the ulcerative type. The lesions had violet overhanging borders, a pustular base, and ulcerating skin with signs of acute inflammation. The underlying cause is believed to be a defective immune response. Wound care plus anti-inflammatory agents and immune system modulators constitute the treatment found to be most effective. Further surgery can worsen the outcome.

▶ Often these patients are placed on prolonged antibiotics without improvement. Because it is an immune process, this makes sense. Therefore, alertness to a nonantibiotic responsive wound should trigger the suspicion of a pyoderma gangrenosum. The mystery is why would a patient with no previous history or immune deficiency develop this process after abdominoplasty?

**P. W. McKinney, MD, CM**

---

**Ten Years of Outpatient Abdominoplasties: Safe and Effective**
Stevens WG, Spring MA, Stoker DA, et al (private practice, Marina Del Rey, CA; private practice, Madison, WI; private practice, Scottsdale, AZ; et al)
*Aesthetic Surg J* 27:269-275, 2007

---

*Background.*—Abdominoplasty is one of the top five cosmetic surgery procedures performed in the United States. Traditionally performed in a hospital setting, more recently procedures are being done in outpatient facilities. The complication and revision rates of patients having outpatient abdominoplasty were compared to the data previously published for in-hospital procedures.

*Methods.*—A retrospective chart review looked at 519 consecutive abdominoplasty procedures performed at an outpatient surgery facility between 1996 and 2006. The average follow-up was 4.3 years, with a range from 6 months to 10 years. Patients' mean age was 43 years, with a range of 19 to 74 years. The charts were reviewed to determine gender, smoking history, American Society of Anesthesiologists (ASA) risk score, body mass index (BMI), type of procedure, and concurrent procedures accomplished. The complication rates and revision rates were determined, noting specifically deaths, venous thromboembolism events, wound dehiscence, infection, seroma, hematoma, and unacceptable scarring.

*Results.*—Full abdominoplasties and floating or mini-abdominoplasties were performed in 88% and 12%, respectively, of the cases reviewed. Only three patients had an ASA risk score of III; the remaining patients all had ASA risk scores of I or II. Additional procedures were performed in 91% of the patients, with the most common add-on being lipoplasty. The postoperative complications reported most often were seroma (10.6% of patients), unacceptable scarring (7.9%), and superficial wound dehiscence (5.6%). None of the patients died. Revision surgery was required for 52 patients, most commonly for unacceptable abdominal scarring. Women had a significantly higher rate of complications than men. Compared to the data in the literature, the total number of complications did not differ significantly.

*Conclusions.*—The outpatient abdominoplasties proved as safe and effective as those performed in the hospital and reported in the literature. All of the procedures were performed at an accredited outpatient surgery facility.

▶ Elective surgery is shifting away from the hospital setting because of doctor control and better anesthesia, which results in more safety for the patient, not to mention one-third the cost. This is one of many articles of a number of plastic surgery operations that document this. My experience echoes theirs, and changing to a freestanding nonhospital, nonuniversity setting was glorious.

**P. W. McKinney, MD, CM**

---

**Resection of Panniculus Morbidus: A Salvage Procedure with a Steep Learning Curve**
Friedrich JB, Petrov RV, Wiechman Askay SA, et al (Univ of Washington, Seattle, WA)
*Plast Reconstr Surg* 121:108-114, 2008

---

*Background.*—A subset of obese people develop a pannus hanging to the floor. This panniculus morbidus prevents weight loss, as the patient cannot exercise. It prevents hygiene, leading to a profound odor and ultimately results in intertrigo, cellulitis, and/or abdominal ulceration. The only two options are to live/die with it or resect it. Some of these people are otherwise ready for a weight loss program. For this group, resection of the panniculus morbidus may be indicated. The authors reviewed the literature and found the condition has not been addressed in this *Journal* since 1994 and was not considered in the recent supplement on body contouring. In 1998, the authors began resecting panniculus morbidus for this small group. The authors found the learning curve to be profoundly steep, with many wound complications, a finding that is quite in conflict with the literature on the subject, and decided to present their experience.

*Methods.*—The authors conducted a retrospective chart review of 23 patients and collected data on demographics, ambulation, hygiene, technique, complications, and outcome.

*Results.*—The technique of closure evolved as the authors struggled with complications. The current method of closure is three suture layers over four suction drains with a small wound vacuum-assisted closure device at each end of the incision. All patients ultimately healed and found it easier to ambulate and perform hygiene.

*Conclusion.*—Resection of panniculus morbidus is a beneficial salvage procedure for some morbidly obese people, but the learning curve is steep and the current literature is misleading.

▶ I applaud the authors of this study for bringing us this report of their experiences with these very difficult problems. They alluded to the fact that few have recently written about panniculus morbidus, and fewer still have focused on the complications associated with a conceptual simple and straightforward surgical procedure. Not all patients with panniculus morbidus are alike, and it is very difficult to compare patients both within a single study and between different studies. What is needed is a universally agreed upon and accepted system to allow a degree of morbid obesity to be categorized based on variables including, but not limited to, weight of the specimen, ulceration, edema, and comorbid factors including age. I believe the authors' suggestion to treat the lateral-most aspects of the wound with the vacuum-assisted closure (VAC) wound device seems reasonable, and I hope to see their results, with this technique, repeated by others on patients with similar degrees of morbidity. The lay press has recently reported that bariatric bypass surgery for obesity has had a positive effect on the management of Type 2 diabetes mellitus. This type of publicity will unquestionably increase the demand for bypass surgery, and very likely for panniculus reduction.

**S. H. Miller, MD, MPH**

### Back Contouring in Weight Loss Patients
Strauch B, Rohde C, Patel MK, et al (Albert Einstein College of Medicine, New York)
*Plast Reconstr Surg* 120:1692-1696, 2007

*Background.*—Body contouring in the post–bariatric surgery patient has focused predominantly on the resulting tissue excesses of the abdomen, breasts, and arms. The back, however, has not received the same attention and, although the skin folds on the back may sometimes be improved by addressing the previously mentioned areas, the result is usually unsatisfactory and leaves the patient with significant residual excess.

*Methods.*—The senior author (B.S.) has developed a classification system and surgical treatment for the excess back tissue that eliminates these folds.

*Results.*—Modifications of the senior author's techniques of mammaplasty/mastopexy and circumferential abdominoplasty, in addition to direct excision, are used to improve the contour of the back.

*Conclusions.*—Contouring of the back roll deformities seen in post–bariatric surgery patients requires a systematic approach. With this approach, the authors have been able to achieve uniform patient satisfaction with low morbidity. Although patients are left with additional scarring, this tradeoff is accepted by nearly all patients for the dramatic improvement in body contour.

▶ Fat removal offers contour correction if (1) some fat remains between the skin and muscle, or (2) the skin will shrink enough to accommodate the new contour. Direct skin resection is indicated if these criteria are not met but with the price of a scar—as the dorsal skin is thicker than ventral skin and contours less easily. Sometimes aggressive suctioning—the ultrasonic method works best in the fibrous dorsal attachments—offers some improvement, but direct excision is often required if a patient is willing to deal with the scars that are more noticeable in the dorsal tissue than the ventral regions.

**P. W. McKinney, MD, CM**

---

**Components Separation Combined with Abdominal Wall Plication for Repair of Large Abdominal Wall Hernias following Bariatric Surgery**
Borud LJ, Grunwaldt L, Janz B, et al (Harvard Med School)
*Plast Reconstr Surg* 119:1792-1798, 2007

---

*Background.*—Abdominal wall hernias frequently occur after open bariatric surgical procedures. Standard repair with synthetic mesh may be suboptimal, with a recurrence rate as high as 50 percent. Patients often seek hernia repair in conjunction with abdominal body contouring procedures following substantial weight loss.

*Methods.*—In 66 consecutive patients undergoing abdominal surgery after open bariatric surgery, abdominal wall hernias of some size were found in 50 patients. In 65 of these patients, panniculectomy was performed simultaneously. The majority of these hernias could be closed primarily in conjunction with abdominal wall plication [38 of 50 (76 percent)]. In 12 patients (24 percent of hernias), the defects were too large (median, 10.8 cm) or located too close to the xiphoid to permit primary closure without undue tension.

*Results.*—Using a components separation technique, primary fascial closure was achieved in all 12 patients. The technique was modified to include abdominal wall plication above and below the repaired hernia defect and the use of an absorbable mesh onlay. Although these patients had a high rate (50 percent) of minor or major superficial wound complications, all wounds closed, subsequently, without additional operative procedures. Despite the high-risk nature of this group, ventral hernia recurred in only one of 12 patients (8.3 percent) after a median follow-up of 16 months. The single recurrence occurred in one of the two patients with the largest diameter (15 cm) hernias in the series.

*Conclusions.*—The components separation technique, combined with abdominal wall plication was assessed as the preferred technique for the repair of large hernias not amenable to primary repair in the massive weight loss patient, following open bariatric procedures. Because this technique avoids placement of permanent mesh, it is particularly advantageous in the post–bariatric surgery patient at high risk for wound dehiscence and infection.

▶ With the increase in bariatric surgery for the morbidly obese, patients are often left with large amounts of redundant tissue and require/request panniculectomy or abdominoplasty to improve their appearance and overall sense of well-being. At the same time, many of these patients have also developed large ventral hernias, as a result of the bariatric surgical procedure. The authors report on a subset of their patients with abdominal wall hernias after bariatric surgery, which could not be managed by direct closure because the defects were too large and or too close to the xiphoid. Using a technique, originally described by Ramirez et al[1] and modified by these authors, they achieved successful closure in 11 of 12 patients, in spite of a high wound complication rate. One of their modifications was to use absorbable mesh between the cut edges of the external oblique fascia to "maintain" the musculofacial flap in its new position, but no data are offered to assess the validity of this maneuver.

I have had similar experiences with separation of the abdominal wall components to repair large postoperative and posttraumatic abdominal wall hernias. Early in my career, and before gaining confidence in the strength of this approach, I tended to overlay the autologous repair with non-absorbable mesh. Having learned the hard way that this material, not infrequently, became the site of an infection when the almost inevitable wound complication occurred, I quickly abandoned the use of mesh and, instead, used fascia lata if I believed a "belt and suspenders" approach to the hernia repair was necessary. It would be interesting to further study the authors' use of absorbable mesh to determine whether it adds to the success of the procedure and makes a difference in allowing the muscle to scar in a more functional position.

**S. H. Miller, MD, MPH**

*Reference*

1. Ramirez OM, Ruas E, Dellon AL. "Components separation" method for closure of abdominal wall defects: an anatomic and clinical study. *Plast Reconstr Surg.* 1990;86:519.

---

**Gluteal augmentation surgery: indications and surgical management**
Harrison D, Selvaggi G (Mount Vernon Hosp, Northwood, Middlesex, England; Wellington Hosp, London)
*J Plast Reconstr Aesthetic Surg* 60:922-928, 2007

---

*Background.*—The gluteal structures not only provide a cushioning effect during sitting but also function in hip joint extension and maintaining balance. In addition, the gluteal region is an important secondary sexual characteristic and is included in concepts of beauty. Gluteal

augmentation and contour reconstruction has included the use of prosthetic implants, liposuction, and fat grafting. Its indications, techniques,
and outcomes were reviewed.

*Indications.*—The primary reasons for performing gluteal reshaping are
gluteal ptosis, hypoplasia, a combination of these two conditions, gluteus
maximus agenesis, hemiatrophy, asymmetry, and fibrosis and deformation
of the gluteal area after silicone injections. Contour reconstruction may be
performed secondary to human immunodeficiency virus (HIV) syndrome
or long-term bed rest. In all cases the patients must be well-motivated
and psychologically prepared for the procedure. It is essential that the
patient cooperate fully during the postoperative stage, especially avoiding
sleeping on the prosthesis.

*Techniques and Complications.*—The surgical techniques are designed
to augment the area with minimal scarring. In complex cases, combinations of techniques may be required. Successful outcomes are possible
using either a silicone prosthesis in the intramuscular or superficial plane
or liposuction/lipo-injection procedures. Implants are simple and easy to
perform but are foreign materials. Placement above the muscle in the
subcutaneous plane can make them more obvious, and rippling can
develop within 18 months. Placement in the intramuscular plane provides
better protection against trauma but muscle clenching can reveal the prosthesis (Fig 1). Complications include wound infections, rupture of the
gluteal prosthesis, infection, extrusion, and hematoma. In liposuction-
lipo-injection gluteoplasty, large volumes of fat are injected over a period
of several hours. Because considerable absorption occurs, the result can be
unpredictable. Good survival of the injected fat and appropriate liposculp-
ture techniques can yield good results. Considerable experience in fat
injection is recommended for the best outcomes. Two HIV-positive
patients developed infection with *Mycobacterium avium* after their procedures. This possibility is not sufficiently common to contraindicate
surgery.

*Conclusions.*—Both reshaping and contour reconstruction of the gluteal
region are effective approaches for achieving a pleasing gluteal appearance. The principal methods are implant placement, liposuction/lipo-injec-
tion, or a combination of these techniques.

▶ Uncommon surgery in the United States. Note how the authors use the cleft
between the buttocks for entry, which reduces the visibility of the scar as well as
keeping the scar at a distance from the prosthesis. The distance is important as
this reduces the change of extrusion. Also, please note the sizes used (250 to

FIGURE 1.—Example of patient who received silicone implant augmentation for correction of small
volume buttocks. First two pictures on the superior line: Status before surgery. All the other pictures:
Status after surgery. Note the shape of the gluteal area and implant when the patient is asked to clench
the gluteus maximus muscle, in the lowest picture on the left side. (Reprinted from Harrison D, Selvaggi
G: Gluteal augmentation surgery: Indications and surgical management. *J Plast Reconstr Aesthetic Surg.*
2007;60:922-928, with permission from the British Association of Plastic, Reconstructive and Aesthetic
Surgery.)

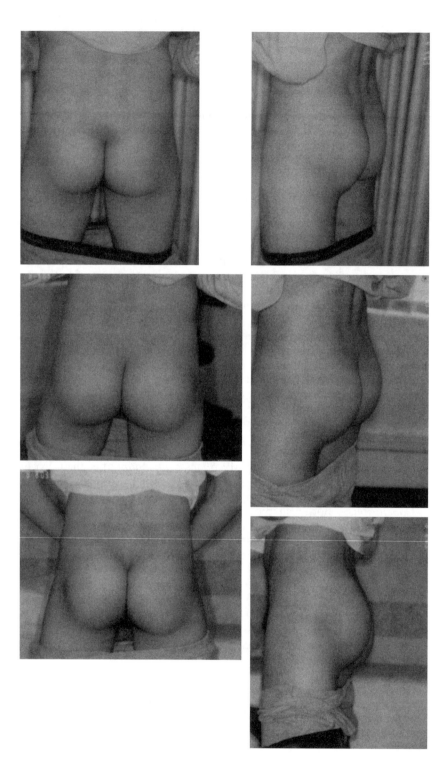

350), and the positioning under the muscle. The placement avoids both positioning and scarring over the ischial tuberosity.

**P. W. McKinney, MD, CM**

# Liposuction, Fat Transfer, and Tissue Fillers

## Plastic surgical options for HIV-associated lipodystrophy
Nelson L, Stewart KJ (St John's Hospital, Livingston, West Lothian, UK)
*J Plast Reconstr Aesthetic Surg* 61:359-365, 2008

With the reported prevalence of HIV-associated lipodystrophy
approaching 80%, this patient group presents an increasing challenge to
plastic surgeons. Based on a literature search conducted using OVID Medline, this review shall describe the various treatment options employed by
plastic surgeons to deal with the problems of fat distribution in patients
suffering from HIV-lipodystrophy, and examine the evidence for each
treatment (Table 2).

▶ The authors of this article have collected, reviewed, and summarized a large
number of articles relating to aesthetic treatment of HIV-associated problems.
The article affords the plastic surgeon a comprehensive compendium of
approaches to these sometimes difficult cases. Of greatest value is the exhaus-
tive bibliography collected by the authors. Once a surgeon selects a technique
for a particular patient, he/she can access appropriate references to obtain more
details about that particular treatment modality, if desired. The authors make no
judgments regarding the preference of one approach over the others—they
simply provide information and references so that surgeons can make their
own decisions in individual cases. The authors do provide some perspectives
about the effectiveness of some of the approaches. There are only a few

TABLE 2.—Therapeutic Options for HIV-Associated Lipodystrophy and Related Metabolic
Complications

◆ Lifestyle changes (reduce saturated fat and cholesterol intake, increase physical activity, cessation of
 smoking)
◆ Change anti-retroviral therapy
◆ Statins
◆ Fibrates
◆ Metformin
◆ Recombinant human growth hormone
◆ Surgical intervention
◆ Plastic surgical options for HIV-associated lipodystrophy

photographic illustrations of cases, so the reader will need to access the primary articles to judge better the effectiveness of a particular approach.

**R. L. Ruberg, MD**

---

### Spontaneous Breast Enlargement following Liposuction of the Abdominal Wall: Does a Link Exist?

van der Lei B, Halbesma G-J, van Nieuwenhoven CA, et al (Med Ctr Leeuwarden, The Netherlands; et al)
*Plast Reconstr Surg* 119:1584-1589, 2007

---

*Background.*—A retrospective study was undertaken to determine the specific incidence of breast enlargement following liposuction of the abdomen (alone or in combination with the flanks), and to compare its effect with a control group of patients who had undergone abdominoplasty only and, where possible, identify corresponding variables.

*Methods.*—Forty-eight of 84 patients (57 percent) who had undergone a tumescent liposuction procedure of at least the abdominal wall and/or flanks and 53 of 104 patients (51 percent) who had undergone abdominoplasty met the entry criteria and formed the study group and the control group, respectively. The medical records were reviewed retrospectively, patient interviews were conducted and, where possible, the patients were examined. Patients who had undergone previous breast or abdominal wall surgery or who had a history of or were breast-feeding at the time of the study were excluded.

*Results.*—In the liposuction group, 23 of the 48 patients (48 percent) reported an increase in their breast size postoperatively. This could objectively be confirmed (by an actual increase of at least one bra cup size) in 19 patients (40 percent). Nine of 19 responders (47 percent) presented with a weight gain of as little as 4 percent of body mass index following liposuction, whereas this was observed in only one of 29 of the nonresponder group (3 percent) ($p < 0.0001$). In the abdominoplasty group, 11 patients (21 percent) claimed to have perceived an increase in breast size, which was objectively confirmed by an increase in bra cup size in six (11 percent) only. Four of the six responders (with an increased cup size) reported a weight gain from as little as 4 percent of body mass index, compared with nine of the remaining 47 patients (19 percent) comprising the nonresponder group ($p < 0.01$).

*Conclusions.*—Liposuction of the abdominal wall and/or flanks is followed by breast enlargement in a significant number of patients (40 percent), a risk that is significantly higher when compared with patients who have undergone abdominoplasty only. Patients should be informed about the possibility and risk of breast enlargement following liposuction of the abdominal wall in particular.

▶ This is now the fourth published study that reports this strange phenomenon. The question is, how do we use this information? One way would be in the form of a warning: Be prepared for your breasts to enlarge after you have abdominal liposuction. But maybe it should be used in a positive way: If you want your breasts to be larger, have abdominal liposuction done. None of these patients had the liposuction done in the effort to increase the size of the breasts. But when this information becomes common knowledge, we can anticipate that there will be patients whose goal is breast enlargement, and who request liposuction principally as a means to achieve this objective. Should we do it? Probably not just for this purpose—this study shows objective enlargement in only 40% of patients.

**R. L. Ruberg, MD**

### A Brief Overview and History of Temporary Fillers: Evolution, Advantages, and Limitations

Fagien S, Klein AW (Univ of California, Los Angeles)
*Plast Reconstr Surg* 120:8S-16S, 2007

Facial soft-tissue augmentation by injection has become increasingly popular as a minimally invasive option for patients seeking cosmetic facial enhancement. Surgical rejuvenation procedures of the face often relate to a less than comprehensive solution to many of the changes that occur with age. Indeed, the surgical "lift," while providing the opportunity for soft-tissue repositioning, often fails to provide volumetric restoration to the face that is lost with aging. Appreciating the necessity of replacing depleted soft tissue has allowed for a more comprehensive approach to total facial rejuvenation. Hundreds of filling agents are available worldwide, and the enormity of options has led to confusion about which agents work best, where, and why. The vast array of available soft-tissue filling agents can be distilled into two simple categories: nonpermanent and permanent. In this article, the authors mostly limit their discussion, consistent with the mission of this supplement, to the evolution of nonpermanent filling agents, providing a rationale for their emergence and their individual use.

▶ Reports of the use of fillers in cosmetic surgery are plentiful, but virtually all are anecdotal, short-term studies that rarely, if ever, prospectively compare end results in a blinded dispassionate fashion, and frequently downplay complications and negative results. The present article, by Faigen and Klein, is a worthwhile article to review, as a starting point, for one's personal review of the historical and current literature regarding tissue fillers for cosmetics. One must do so, however, with the knowledge that both of the authors are investigators and consultants to many of the companies manufacturing these materials. This is, certainly, an area of medical practice that is "crying out" for some semblance of ordered prospective studies, dictated by agreed upon technical protocols as to sites for injection, depth, etc, evaluative "blinded" outcome assessments, documentation of duration, and costs. It would also be very interesting to see how well these fillers disguise the soft-tissue deformity when using their muscles of facial expression.

**S. H Miller, MD, MPH**

---

### Collagenous Microbeads as a Scaffold for Tissue Engineering with Adipose-Derived Stem Cells
Rubin JP, Bennett JM, Doctor JS, et al (Univ of Pittsburgh, PA; Duquesne Univ, Pittsburgh, PA; McGowan Inst for Regenerative Medicine, Pittsburgh, PA)
*Plast Reconstr Surg* 120:414-424, 2007

---

*Background.*—Standard approaches to soft-tissue reconstruction include autologous tissue flaps and alloplastic implants. Both of these approaches have disadvantages, including donor-site morbidity, implant migration, and foreign body reaction. Autologous fat transplantation, with a minimally invasive cannula harvest, has lower donor-site morbidity than tissue flaps do, but there is an unpredictable degree of resorption of the transplanted fat over time. Adipose-derived stem cells isolated from harvested fat are better able to withstand the mechanical trauma from the suction cannula and may allow for improved cell survival and generation of new fat tissue after transfer to another anatomic site. The authors hypothesized that porous collagenous microbeads (CultiSphers; Sigma, St. Louis, Mo.) could be useful as injectable cell delivery vehicles for adipose-derived stem cells. This strategy would allow induction of differentiation ex vivo and precise placement of cells and scaffold in a tissue bed. The objective of this study was to assess the ability of the stem cells to proliferate and differentiate on these microbeads.

*Methods.*—Adipose-derived stem cells were isolated from discarded human adipose tissue and cultured on porous collagenous microbeads in a stirred bioreactor (spinner flask). The cells attached and proliferated on the microbeads and maintained high viability over several weeks of culture.

*Results.*—When exposed to adipogenic or osteogenic medium, the cells differentiated into adipocytes and osteoblasts, respectively, while attached to the microbeads.

*Conclusion.*—Collagenous microbeads are a favorable scaffold for adipose-derived stem cells, allowing ex vivo proliferation and differentiation on particles that are small enough to be injected.

▶ When collagenous microbeads were used as a scaffold, fat-derived adipose stem cells proliferated, and the authors believe they will prove useful for soft tissue reconstruction. When compared with other technology,[1] the cell-seeded microbeads can be injected into the site where fill is needed and allow immediate exposure of the stem cells to interstitial nutrient fluid. It still remains to be seen that this technology will, in fact, produce adipose tissue that predictably survives. Nonetheless, the technology is potentially very exciting and should be followed carefully for new developments.

**S. H. Miller, MD, MPH**

*Reference*

1. Stosich MS, Mao JJ. Adipose tissue engineering from human adult stem cells: clinical implications in plastic and reconstructive surgery. *Plast Reconstr Surg.* 2007; 119:71-83.

---

**Autologous Fat Transfer for Facial Recontouring: Is There Science behind the Art?**
Kaufman MR, Miller TA, Huang C, et al (Univ of California, Los Angeles)
*Plast Reconstr Surg* 119:2287-2296, 2007

---

*Background.*—Clinical use of autologous fat grafts for facial soft-tissue augmentation has grown in popularity in the plastic surgery community, despite a perceived drawback of unpredictable results.

*Methods.*—The authors' review of the literature and their current techniques of autologous fat transfer focused on (1) the donor site, (2) aspiration methods, (3) local anesthesia, (4) centrifugation and washing, (5) exposure to cold and air, (6) addition of growth factors, (7) reinjection methods, and (8) longevity of fat grafts.

*Results.*—Clinical experience and basic science data showed a slight preference for the following: harvesting abdominal fat with "nontraumatic," blunt cannula technique, preparation by means of centrifugation without washing or addition of growth factors, and immediate injection of small amounts of fat by means of multiple passes. Quantitative evidence of clinical fat survivability and predictability of volume restoration does not exist, yet reports of patient satisfaction with this procedure do. Clinicians report the need for revisionary procedures to optimize results.

*Conclusions.*—Although there is an increased trend in replacement of soft-tissue volume with autologous fat transfer, the literature fails to provide definitive evidence of fat survival. A large-scale clinical assessment, using three-dimensional volumetric imaging, would provide useful outcome data.

▶ This is a very good article reviewing the current state and knowledge about fat transfer for facial recontouring. By and large, this appears to be an often-used technique by many plastic surgeons and other physicians, with little in the way of hard evidence to document the most appropriate processes to use for it to be effective. Whether the fat actually survives, and if it does not, what is the basis for patient and physician satisfaction? Some of the more exciting work in this regard has come about through engineering adipose tissue using mesenchymal stem cells.[1]

The authors conclude, and I agree, that it should be possible using 3-dimensional volumetric imaging, and perhaps cell labeling to document effectiveness and whether or not fat survives. However, such studies will require carefully constructed protocols and collaborations at institutions with the expertise and capability to initiate and complete such studies. Failure to study this procedure and document the results clearly and appropriately leads many to question its effectiveness and efficiency.

**S. H. Miller, MD, MPH**

*Reference*

1. Stosich MS, Mao JJ. Adipose tissue engineering from human adult stem cells: clinical implications in plastic and reconstructive surgery. *Plast Reconstr Surg.* 2007; 119:71-83.

---

**Facial Augmentation with Core Fat Graft: A Preliminary Report**
Guyuron B, Majzoub RK (Case Western Reserve Univ, Cleveland, OH)
*Plast Reconstr Surg* 120:295-302, 2007

---

*Background.*—Facial rejuvenation with autologous fat has the advantage of replacing or augmenting tissue with like tissue. The results of injected fat are unpredictable because of cellular trauma and other factors. Excised whole or en bloc fat grafting has been shown, experimentally, to have a greater percentage of adipocyte survival when compared with blunt cannula delivery techniques. En bloc grafting, however, requires an incision for the harvesting and placement of the fat graft with visible scars. A novel, less traumatic cylinder core fat harvest and delivery technique for facial augmentation with minimal incisional access is reported here.

*Methods.*—Twenty-six facial augmentation procedures were performed involving the malar area, buccal area, lips, nasolabial folds, and mental region. Fat transfer volume ranged between 1 and 4 cc per site. In this report, 16 patients' results were documented 6 to 16 months postoperatively (mean follow-up time, 9.5 months) with a postoperative questionnaire and photographs.

*Results.*—Social recovery for patients was short, with a recovery time of 2 to 20 days (mean, 10.91 days). There were no procedure-related complications at the fat harvest or recipient graft sites. The need for overcorrection was minimal. Graft maintenance during the average follow-up at 9.5 months appeared excellent and without appreciable volume loss. The mean patient satisfaction score was 7.64 ± 2.97 on a scale of 0 to 10.

*Conclusions.*—The authors' preliminary results have demonstrated that this technique is effective and highly predictable. The surgical time was short, and patient recovery time has been significantly reduced, compared with recovery time after other fat injection techniques.

▶ This intriguing technique follows the basic surgical principle—less trauma equals greater tissue survival. Taking of core fat with a tuberculin syringe does not require any special instrumentation either. This technique may be just right for the nasolabial folds.

**P. W. Mckinney, MD, CM**

---

**Introduction of an Easy Technique for Purification and Injection of Autogenous Free Fat Parcels in Correcting of Facial Contour Deformities**
Hu S, Zhang H, Feng Y, et al (Chinese Academy of Med Sciences, Beijing, China)
*Ann Plast Surg* 58:602-607, 2007

---

*Background.*—Facial contour deformities usually result from congenital abnormalities, trauma, and the aging process. All depressions in the face, including glabella wrinkles and mild retrogression of chins, fall in this category. Local injection of autogenous fat parcels has been introduced for correction of these facial deformities for almost 20 years.

*Method.*—Using common materials (gauzes and cotton sticks), a simple technique was used, by us, to purify syringe-suctioned fat parcels followed by a multilayered injection of the purified fat tissue into implantation sites to treat the facial contour deformities in 152 sites of 50 cases with successful outcomes.

*Results.*—Thirty-nine sites, in 17 cases, were followed up from 13 months to 37 months (average, 22.8 months). The injected fat parcels deposited successfully, and the increasing volume maintained well. The impact factors on the successful deposit of the injected fat parcels included the extent of mechanical injuries to the fat cells during liposuction and lipoinjection, application of the purification procedure, and postsurgery immobilization as well as the blood-nourishing situation of recipient sites. Postoperative complications included undercorrection, overcorrection, small fat mass, unevenness, or irregularity.

*Conclusion.*—The introduced purification and injection techniques provided a comparative simple, and reliable method, in facial recontouring treatment. The local volume could be increased successfully by means of controlling the influencing factors of fat parcel deposit.

▶ This is an interesting study from colleagues in China, outlining their preferred techniques for harvesting, preparing, and using fat "parcels" to correct facial contour deformities. Key to their approach was harvesting with small, blunt cannulas, purifying the fat "parcels" by separating the suctioned material into components, and by only using the fat "parcel" for injection. The latter was performed in layers through large bore syringes. Results were said to be quite good, but undercorrection, was very common, especially in mobile tissues, and results were less than optimal for deformities caused by trauma, infection, or operation. Documentation of fat survival was not reported.

**S. H. Miller, MD, MPH**

**Bioartificial Dermal Substitute: A Preliminary Report on Its Use for the Management of Complex Combat-Related Soft Tissue Wounds**
Helgeson MD, Potter BK, Evans KN, et al (Walter Reed Army Med Ctr, Washington, DC)
*J Orthop Trauma* 21:394-399, 2007

*Objective.*—To report our institutional experience with the use of a bioartificial dermal substitute (Integra) combined with subatmospheric pressure [vacuum-assisted closure (VAC)] dressings followed by delayed split-thickness skin grafting for management of complex combat-related soft tissue wounds secondary to blast injuries.
*Design.*—Retrospective review of patients treated December 2004 through November 2005.
*Setting.*—Military treatment facility.
*Patients/Participants.*—Integra grafting was performed 18 times in 16 wounds at our institution. Indications for Integra placement were wounds not amenable to simple split-thickness skin grafting, specifically those with substantial exposed bone and/or tendon.
*Intervention.*—Patients underwent an average of 8.5 irrigation and debridement procedures and concurrent VAC dressings prior to placement of the Integra. Following Integra grafting, all patients were managed with VAC dressings, changed every 3 to 4 days at the bedside or in clinic, with subsequent split-thickness skin grafting an average of 19 days later.
*Main Outcome Measurements.*—The mechanism and date of injury, size of residual soft tissue deficit, indication for Integra placement, number of irrigation and debridement procedures prior to Integra placement, days from injury to Integra placement, days from Integra placement to split-thickness skin grafting, and clinical outcome were recorded.
*Results.*—Integra placement and subsequent skin grafting was successful in achieving durable and cosmetic definitive coverage in 15 of 16 wounds with two of these patients requiring repeat Integra application. Two patients with difficult VAC dressing placement had early Integra graft failure but successfully healed following repeated Integra application and skin grafting.
*Conclusions.*—Bioartificial dermal substitute grafting, when coupled with subatmospheric dressing management and delayed split-thickness skin grafting, is an effective technique for managing complex combat-related soft tissue wounds with exposed tendon. This can potentially lessen the need for local rotational or free flap coverage.

▶ First, I must give the caveat that I am on the Integra speaker's bureau. I think this article provides another excellent use for this product as a possible long-term solution for complex soft tissue wounds. If a wound can be debrided to predictably healthy tissue, Integra may act as a temporary cover, creating a neo-dermis, which can then be grafted for a long-term stable wound closure. The vacuum-assisted closure (VAC), of course, helpful in this setting of an acutely inflamed and edematous wound. The Integra should be meshed to facilitate drainage through the matrix. For those of you who do not routinely mesh Integra, I believe that this product will be available off the shelf in the meshed version soon. The final results with this protocol works make me question, whether or not this algorithm can be successful in patients with exposed fractures. Clearly, more study is needed to determine if this is safe in other situations than the immediate postcasualty setting. Until then, we do not know the safety of this algorithm.

**W. L. Garner, MD**

## A Two-Stage Phase I Trial of Evolence[30] Collagen for Soft-Tissue Contour Correction
Monstrey SJ, Pitaru S, Hamdi M, et al (Univ Hosp Gent, Belgium; Tel Aviv Univ, Israel; Sheba Med Ctr, Ramat-Gan, Israel; et al)
*Plast Reconstr Surg* 120:303-311, 2007

*Background.*—The ideal dermal filler should be nonpermanent, but with a durable effect, lasting between 1 and 2 years, which is not the case with the resorbable fillers that are currently available. Evolence[30] is a new, porcine-derived collagen gel based on the Glymatrix cross-linking technology, which results in a more natural and longer-lasting collagen product.

*Methods.*—In this first clinical trial of Evolence[30] (30 mg/ml), the safety and efficacy of this new filler were tested and compared with those of Zyplast (bovine cross-linked) collagen, after treatment of nasolabial folds in 12 volunteers. Safety assessments included two hypersensitivity tests, physical examination of injections sites, punch biopsies for histopathology, adverse events, and blood sample analysis. The seven-grade, validated Modified Fitzpatrick Wrinkle Scale was used by three independent blinded assessors to evaluate efficacy.

*Results.*—No treatment-related adverse events were reported. Only transient erythema was observed in both treated sides, and there were no abnormal laboratory findings. None of the sera contained immunoglobulin (Ig) M, IgA, or IgE antibodies against porcine collagen at any time during the study. Initially, Evolence[30] and Zyplast improved wrinkle severity to a similar extent. However, in an average follow-up of 18 months, assessment by the blinded assessors showed that the treatment effect on the Evolence[30]-treated side was superior in 9 of the 11 participants who were treated ($p = 0.022$).

*Conclusions.*—Evolence[30] is a new, porcine-derived collagen product, based on the Glymatrix cross-linking technology, that enables a safe and effective correction of the nasolabial folds. This correction lasts significantly longer than that with Zyplast.

▶ I have to look beyond the name of the material, which is more marketing than science. Evolence does fulfill a prime criterion for any injectable; that is, it is either easily removable or it will be gradually absorbed. However, there are many articles regarding permanent fillers, but if they need removal they are dangerous. I know that small droplets and small quantities offer small chance of complications, but small quantities do not always happen, especially in inexperienced hands. A filler is an easy solution to small nasal defects with no potential for sharp edges. However, we must consider the material used very carefully. Some of us recall the story of paraffin where early in the 20th century an entire textbook on plastic surgery was devoted to injectable paraffin with excellent photographs using nasal profiles as examples. Paraffin was used in the breasts, limbs, cheeks, etc for over 50 years until its sclerotic effect became obvious. There are many good materials available today that are unfortunately printed in our scientific journals with marketing names rather than scientific ones, making objective evaluation difficult. As a common denominator, the safest ones will be those that gradually dissolve or can easily be removed in unusual circumstances.

**P. W. McKinney, MD, CM**

### Calcium Hydroxylapatite (Radiesse) for Correction of the Mid- and Lower Face: Consensus Recommendations
Graivier MH, Bass LS, Busso M, et al (New York Univ School of Medicine)
*Plast Reconstr Surg* 120:55S-66S, 2007

Restoring volume in the middle and lower portions of the face is becoming an indispensable component of modern facial rejuvenation. Radiesse (BioForm Medical, San Mateo, Calif.) is an injectable filler material composed of synthetic calcium hydroxylapatite microspheres (30 percent) suspended in an aqueous carrier gel (70 percent). At present, Radiesse is indicated in the United States for correction of moderate to deep nasolabial folds and for correction of the signs of facial fat loss (lipoatrophy) in people with human immunodeficiency virus. Its off-label use in other facial aesthetic indications is widely reported in the literature. The ability of Radiesse to provide immediate and durable effects has fueled interest in its use for expanded aesthetic applications, particularly in the middle and lower face. The authors' consensus panel, consisting of a cross-section of experts in plastic surgery, facial plastic surgery, and dermatology, was convened to review the scientific literature and compare clinical experiences regarding the use of calcium hydroxylapatite. This report describes the characteristic effects of aging in the middle and lower face and reviews the composition of calcium hydroxylapatite, its safety and durability, and its appropriate use in a variety of facial applications, including nasolabial folds, correction of human immunodeficiency virus–associated lipoatrophy, augmentation of the malar, submalar, and zygomatic regions, and correction of oral commissure defects, marionette lines, and prejowl sulcus. Recommendations for Radiesse use in each area, including anesthesia, and injection techniques are provided. Measures for enhancing patient comfort, anticipating and minimizing potential complications, and optimizing aesthetic results are also discussed.

▶ Hurrah! A scientific article on fillers using a scientific name. Why is this important? It tells us that the article was probably written for the physician's judgment instead of the publicist's (well, almost, because we are saturated later with its public relations name). The material is slowly absorbed (Fig 1 in the original article), does not form granuloma (so far), and does not calcify (so far). Fillers offer in-office corrections and, therefore, offer tremendous appeal to the patient, but the materials require constant scrutiny as to their long-term effects.[1]

**P. W. McKinney, MD, CM**

*Reference*

1. de Lacerda DA, Zancanaro P. Filler rhinoplasty. *Dermatol Surg.* 2007;33: S207-S212.

# 6 Breast

## General

**Fat Grafting to the Breast Revisited: Safety and Efficacy**
Coleman SR, Saboeiro AP (New York Univ)
*Plast Reconstr Surg* 119:775-785, 2007

*Background.*—A 1987 American Society of Plastic and Reconstructive Surgeons position paper predicted that fat grafting would compromise breast cancer detection and should therefore be prohibited. However, there is no evidence that fat grafting to breasts is less safe than any other form of breast surgery. As discussions of fat grafting to the breast are surfacing all over the world, it is time to reexamine the opinions of the 1987 American Society of Plastic and Reconstructive Surgeons position paper.

*Methods.*—This is a retrospective examination of 17 breast procedures performed using fat grafting from 1995 to 2000. Indications included micromastia, postaugmentation deformity, tuberous breast deformity, Poland's syndrome, and postmastectomy reconstruction deformities. The technique used was the Coleman method of fat grafting, which attempts to minimize trauma and place grafted fat in small aliquots at many levels.

*Results.*—All women had a significant improvement in their breast size and/or shape postoperatively and all had breasts that were soft and natural in appearance and feel. Postoperative mammograms identified changes one would expect after any breast procedure.

*Conclusions.*—Given these results and reports of other plastic surgeons, free fat grafting should be considered as an alternative or adjunct to breast augmentation and reconstruction procedures. It is time to end the discrimination created by the 1987 position paper and judge fat grafting to the breast with the same caution and enthusiasm as any other useful breast procedure.

▶ This article is published with a dual purpose: (1) To show that fat grafting for breast augmentation and contouring is effective, and (2) To influence the American Society of Plastic Surgeons to change its official position regarding the safety and suitability of fat grafting to the breast. I am convinced of the validity of the first point (Fig 2 in the original article). Dr. Coleman uses a very tedious and time-consuming technique to achieve his good results, and I am not sure whether his personal approach is necessary (ie, can the same result be achieved with larger fat bolus injections over less time?), but it certainly works. As far as the second objective is concerned, at the time of this writing there has been no change in the official policy of the ASPS-so far.

**R. L. Ruberg, MD**

---

**Congenital Breast Deformity Reconstruction Using Perforator Flaps**
Gautam AK, Allen RJ Jr, LoTempio MM, et al (LSU, New Orleans, LA; Med Univ of South Carolina, Charleston)
*Ann Plast Surg* 58:353-358, 2007

---

*Background.*—Congenital breast deformities, such as Poland syndrome, unilateral congenital hypoplasia, tuberous breast anomaly, and amastia pose a challenging plastic surgical dilemma. The majority of patients are young, healthy individuals who seek esthetic restoration of their breast deformities. Currently, both implant and autologous reconstructive techniques are used. This study focuses on our experience with congenital breast deformity patients who underwent reconstruction using a perforator flap.

*Methods.*—From 1994 to 2005, a retrospective chart review was performed on women who underwent breast reconstruction using perforator flaps to correct congenital breast deformities and asymmetry. Patient age, breast deformity type, perforator flap type, flap volume, recipient vessels, postoperative complications, revisions, and esthetic results were determined.

*Results.*—Over an 11-year period, 12 perforator flaps were performed. All cases were for unilateral breast deformities. The patients ranged from 16 to 43 years of age. Six patients had undergone previous correctional surgeries. Eight (n = 8) flaps were used for correction of Poland syndrome and its associated chest wall deformities. Four (n = 4) flaps were used for correction of unilateral breast hypoplasia. In all cases, the internal mammary vessels were the recipient vessels of choice. No flaps were lost. No vein grafts were used. All patients were discharged on the fourth postoperative day. Complications encountered included seroma, hematoma, and nipple malposition. Revisional surgery was performed in 30% of the cases. Esthetic results varied from poor to excellent.

*Conclusions.*—Perforator flaps are an acceptable choice for patients with congenital breast deformities seeking autologous breast reconstruction. Deep inferior epigastric artery (DIEP), or superficial inferior epigastric artery (SIEA) flaps, are performed when adequate abdominal tissue is available; however, many young patients have inadequate abdominal tissue, thus a GAP flap can be used. Perforator flaps are a safe, reliable surgical technique. In the properly selected patient, donor-site morbidity and functional compromise are minimized, improved self-esteem is noted, postoperative pain is decreased, and excellent long-term esthetic results can be achieved.

▶ The results of this approach are generally quite acceptable (see Fig 1 in the original article), although the revision rate of 30% is certainly significant. I find that lesser degrees of deformity (usually with minor degrees of asymmetry) are quire amenable to implant techniques. On the other hand, more significant deformities of the breast, and (especially) more noticeable, abnormalities of the bony and soft tissue chest structures require autogenous tissue reconstructive techniques. The perforator flap is 1 (but not the only) applicable method of autogenous reconstruction for congenital breast deformities.

**R. L. Ruberg, MD**

---

**Reconstruction of Total Absence of the Breast**
Garcia O Jr (Univ of Miami, FL)
*Ann Plast Surg* 58:12-17, 2007

---

*Background.*—Complete absence of the breast is extremely rare. It occurs as bilateral absence plus congenital ectodermal defect, unilateral absence, or bilateral absence alone. Breast absence is often accompanied by anomalies of other body structures. The reconstructive options include prostheses, staged reconstruction, subpectoral tissue expansion plus implants, and pedicled transverse rectus abdominis myocutaneous (TRAM) flaps. A case of complete absence of the breast with significant deformities was reported.

> *Case Report.*—Woman, 31, had complete absence of the left breast. She had two children who had no breast deformities and there was no family history. Her marriage was stable, and she was well-adjusted to her congenital anomaly. Physical examination revealed left chest wall deformity with complete absence of the breast, underlying muscles, and ribs plus ptosis of the right breast. Three-dimensional spiral computed tomography (CT) and axial CT showed the defects well. She was seeking surgery to create a left breast mound and symmetry with her right breast. The TRAM flap was chosen to recreate the breast mound in a staged reconstruction approach.
>
> In the first stage, the left breast mound was created and a right mastopexy was performed. The skin overlying the pleura was deep-ithelialized, and the contralateral fascial-sparing pedicled TRAM flap was transferred over the defect. Extra soft-tissue coverage over the pleura was accomplished by using a significant part of the muscle underlying the flap. Shaping and tailoring were accomplished on the abdomen before the flap was transferred. The right

and left breast mounds were fairly symmetric in volume and shape once these procedures were accomplished.

Stage 2, 4 mouths later, consisted of nipple reconstruction, minor revisions of scars, and shaping of the flap. Most of the flap shaping was accomplished via liposuction.

In stage 3, 4 months later, intradermal pigmentation of the reconstructed left nipple-areola was addressed. In addition, the upper pole and left inframammary fold underwent further liposuction.

Six months later the final stage was accomplished. Suction-assisted lipectomy of the right anterior axillary fold and fat grafting of the deficient left anterior axillary fold were performed to achieve a more symmetric appearance. Three months after the final revisions, or about 15 months after beginning the reconstruction, the process was complete.

*Conclusions.*—Staged breast reconstruction can achieve good symmetry of volume and shape for women with complete congenital absence of the breast. The anomaly is rare and presents with significant heterogeneity in both inheritance and clinical appearance. The TRAM flap was used in the reported case, with the final results achieved 15 months after beginning the process.

▶ The value of this article is 2-fold. First of all, it demonstrates an excellent result of total breast and associated chest wall bony and soft tissue reconstruction using a transverse rectus abdominis myocutaneous (TRAM) flap plus additional ancillary procedures. Secondly, it effectively summarizes the literature related to total absence of the breast and provides a usable classification system, which is based on previous work by Trier.[1] I have personally treated many patients with varying degrees of hypoplasia of the breast, some also with accompanying muscle hypoplasia (Poland's anomaly), but only 1 case of total absence of the breast. The result produced by this author using autogenous tissue reconstructive techniques is clearly better than the result I achieved many years ago using implant techniques alone.

**R. L. Ruberg, MD**

*Reference*

1. Trier WC. Complete breast absence: case report and review of the literature. *Plast Reconstr Surg.* 1965;36:431-439.

## The tuberous breast revisited

Pacifico MD, Kang NV (Mount Vernon Hosp, Northwood, Middlesex, England)
*J Plast Reconstr Aesthetic Surg* 60:455-464, 2007

*Background.*—The tuberous breast presents a problem for which many surgical solutions have been described. Current teaching describes how the tuberous breast deformity is the result of skin shortage, as well as herniation of breast tissue through the nipple–areola complex. However, through careful clinical observation, we now believe that the only abnormality present is herniation of breast tissue through the nipple–areola complex.

*Methods.*—Using this principle, we have refined a one-stage surgical procedure that can be used to correct any type of tuberous breast deformity. Since 2001, we have performed our technique on a series of 13 tuberous breasts of widely varying appearances in eight patients (age 17–24 years), with a follow up varying between 3 and 56 months. Our new understanding of the tuberous breast deformity has also made it possible to develop an objective, reproducible method for defining the tuberous breast based on the degree of areola herniation.

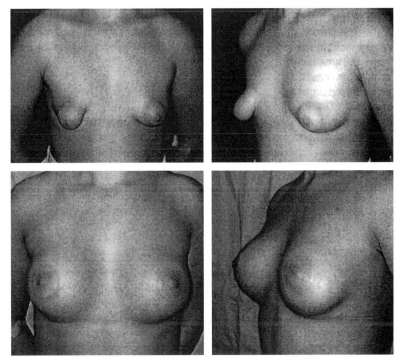

FIGURE 5.—Pre- and postoperative appearances of patient 1 at 56 months. Bilateral tuberous breast deformities – 170 cc and 230 cc high profile round cohesive gel implants used for the left and right breasts, respectively. (Courtesy of Pacifico MD & Kang NV. The tuberous breast revisited. *J Plast Reconstr Aesthetic Surg.* 2007;60:455-464, Reprinted with permission from British Association of Plastic, Reconstructive and Aesthetic Surgeons.)

*Results.*—All patients reported high levels of satisfaction with the procedure. Assessment of the results, by an independent panel of attending surgeons, showed all results to be good/excellent. Moreover, the results have improved with time, and no revisions have been needed. Our method of defining the tuberous breast (based on the ratio of areola herniation:areola diameter) enabled us to identify a cut-off to decide (objectively) when a breast was tuberous. This allowed us to anticipate when an areola reduction/tightening procedure would be necessary to avoid a 'double-bubble' deformity.

*Conclusion.*—We propose a one-stage surgical procedure, which is applicable to all degrees of tuberous breast deformity. The results appear to confirm our theory that the only abnormality present in the tuberous breast is herniation of breast tissue through the nipple–areola complex. In patients with small breasts and a tuberous deformity, correction of the herniation changes the tuberous breast into a simple hypoplastic breast. The volume deficit can then be corrected by augmentation (if desired by the patient). In patients with sufficient breast volume, correction of the herniation, alone, will correct the deformity (Fig 5).

▶ Not everyone would agree with the authors that the only deformity of the tuberous breast is the nipple/areola "herniation." Many people still believe that some degree of constriction of the base of the breast contributes to the deformity and must be corrected. Whether the constriction is present or not is debatable, but the quality of the results, shown in the article, is not (see Fig 5). My own approach is to address the herniation, and if I am adding an implant or expanding, I also release the base of the breast because I am already in the proper (subglandular) plane. The added time and risk for the latter step is minimal.

**R. L. Ruberg, MD**

# Mastopexy and Reduction

### Dermabond Skin Closures for Bilateral Reduction Mammaplasties: A Review of 255 Consecutive Cases
Scott GR, Carson CL, Borah GL (Univ of Medicine and Dentistry of New Jersey)
*Plast Reconstr Surg* 120:1460-1465, 2007

*Background.*—2-Octyl cyanoacrylate (Dermabond; Ethicon, Inc., Somerville, N.J.) has been available as a skin closure alternative or adjunct since 1997. The purpose of this study was to review a large series of 255 consecutive bilateral reduction mammaplasty patients to evaluate the safety and efficacy of Dermabond for these procedures.

*Methods.*—A review was undertaken of 255 consecutive bilateral reduction mammaplasties performed by a single surgeon from 1999 to 2005 with Dermabond used for skin closure. This series of patients was compared with an earlier review by the same surgeon of 415 consecutive bilateral reduction mammaplasties using standard layered sutured skin closures.

*Results.*—Dermabond was associated with decreased operative times compared with the sutured closures (93 minutes compared with 118 minutes; 25 minutes or 20 percent less time). The rates for minor wound dehiscence (1.18 percent), major wound dehiscence (0.78), hypertrophic scar revisions (2.75 percent), and cellulitis (2.75 percent) were all lower in the Dermabond group, but these differences were not statistically significant.

*Conclusions.*—Dermabond is a safe and effective means of skin closure for bilateral reduction mammaplasties. Shortened operative times can lead to economic health cost savings. Patient discomfort is minimized and postoperative care is simplified.

▶ The use of dermal adhesive has increasing popularity as speed in the operating room takes on more and more importance. This investigation is not a prospective, randomized study, so one could criticize the validity of the conclusions. The "controls" are historical (ie, a previously-done group of patients). Nevertheless, I think the conclusion is probably useful—gluing the skin works just as well as, and takes less time than, intradermal sutures for closure. Some of my colleagues have now combined several new approaches to achieve even more significant reduction of surgery time (eg, deep-barbed sutures and superficial dermal adhesive). The result is even less intraoperative time. One factor needs more attention when considering these techniques—cost. Some of our community surgeons will use 1 closure method when doing hospital-based cases and another when working in their own surgical facilities. The decision is based on the cost of the supplies (eg, suture type, dermal adhesive). When they are paying for every single aspect of the procedure, they will tend to use the least expensive, yet still perfectly effective, method.

**R. L. Ruberg, MD**

## The Versatility of the Superomedial Pedicle with Various Skin Reduction Patterns

Davison SP, Mesbahi AN, Ducic I, et al (Georgetown Univ Hosp, Washington, DC)

*Plast Reconstr Surg* 120:1466-1476, 2007

*Background.*—The inferior pedicle technique remains one of the most commonly used techniques in breast reduction surgery, despite lengthy operating times, poor nipple sensation, and bottoming-out over time. The superomedial pedicle in reduction mammaplasty has previously been described using limited incision patterns. This study evaluated the safety and reliability of the superomedial pedicle with various skin reduction patterns and compared the surgical time with the inferior pedicle technique.

*Methods.*—A total of 279 superomedial breast reductions were reviewed over a 6-year period, representing the transition period from inferior pedicle to superomedial pedicle techniques of three attending surgeons. Among these reductions, 215 had complete records and were included in the data analysis. The remaining 64 records were evaluated for viability of the nipple-areola complex. Assessments included skin pattern markings, average size of reduction, average body mass index, and complications. Risk factors and patient comorbidities were also recorded.

*Results.*—There were no cases of nipple loss in the series. The overall complication rate was 18 percent; patients' average body mass index was 29. The revision rate for contour or scar improvement was 4 percent. A statistically significant reduction in operating time of 41 minutes ($p = 0.0001$) was seen in comparison with the inferior pedicle reduction.

*Conclusions.*—The superomedial dermoglandular pedicle is a safe and reliable technique for reduction mammaplasty. Its versatility allows for reproducible results in a broad range of patients with various skin excision patterns. Use of the superomedial pedicle provides consistent results with respect to breast contour, nipple viability, and lasting superomedial fullness, and saves operating time compared with the inferior pedicle technique.

▶ This is a report of a very large series of patients undergoing breast reduction surgery in a single institution, using superomedial pedicles ala Findley-Hall[1] rather than inferiorly based pedicles. The authors conclude that the use of this technique is faster, safer, more aesthetic than the inferior pedicle technique, and also easier to teach. The technique is by no means new and variations of it have been described since 1975, yet the inferior dermal pedicle remains the most popular technique for reduction mammaplasty. Perhaps 1 reason is related to the inconsistent results and difficulty in tailoring the breast with some of the earlier superior pedicle techniques.[2] The authors report that in their hands, most of the objections to the use of the superomedial flap have been overcome; however, they do not discuss the learning curve when first adopting this technique, nor do they actually compare the results with a contemporaneously performed inferior pedicle series. The follow-up is too short to state that the degree of superomedial fullness is lasting and there is less bottoming out than with the inferior pedicle technique. In my view, the inferior descent of the breast/bottoming out is a function of several issues rather than entirely the location of the base of the pedicle. Some of the reasons include the elasticity and weight of the remaining tissues, and the timing of the postoperative assessment. In addition to nipple viability, it would be useful to have data regarding nipple sensibility. Finally, I am concerned with the lack of uniformity in the photographic poses when the arms are clasped behind the body.

Differences in their position and tension can be decided to alter the position and height of the breasts.

**S. H. Miller, MD, MPH**

*References*

1. Hall-Findley J. Vertical breast reduction: New Trends in Reduction Mammaplasty, Seminars. *Plast Surg.* 2004;18:211.
2. Orlando JD, Gurthrie RH Jr. The superomedial dermal pedicle for nipple transposition. *Br J Plast Surg.* 1975;28:42.

**Vertical Scar Reduction Mammaplasty: The Fate of Nipple-Areola Complex Position and Inferior Pole Length**

Ahmad J, Lista F (Univ of Texas Southwestern Med Ctr, Dallas; Trillium Health Ctr, Mississauga, ON, Canada)

*Plast Reconstr Surg* 121:1084-1091, 2008

*Background.*—A major advantage of vertical scar reduction mammaplasty is the improved long-term projection of the breasts. In their experience with more than 1700 cases, the authors have observed the following important trends: Postoperatively, the nipple-areola complex is located higher than one would predict from the preoperative skin markings, and pseudoptosis does not occur. This study was performed to provide objective measurements to confirm these observations.

*Methods.*—Forty-nine consecutive women had the following measurements taken of their right breast preoperatively and on postoperative day 5: distance from the clavicle to the superior border of the nipple-areola complex; the clavicle to the nipple; and the inframammary crease to the inferior border of the nipple-areola complex. Forty-six women were available for follow-up at 4 years, and measurements were repeated.

*Results.*—Compared with preoperative skin markings, the nipple-areola complex was located on average 1.3 cm higher on postoperative day 5 and 1.0 cm higher at 4-year follow-up. The average distance from the inframammary crease to the inferior border of the nipple-areola complex had decreased 0.4 cm at 4-year follow-up.

*Conclusions.*—Compared with preoperative skin markings, the nipple-areola complex was located significantly higher at both early and long-term follow-up. The authors have adjusted their skin marking technique so that the superior border of the nipple-areola complex is marked at the level of the inframammary crease. At 4 years, the distance from the inframammary crease to the inferior border of the nipple-areola complex was significantly shorter, and pseudoptosis did not occur after vertical scar reduction mammaplasty.

▶ This is an important article, but not for the reasons given by the authors. The authors recommend adjusting the position of the nipple areola complex to a somewhat lower level than they had used before because the nipple "rises" after the reduction is completed. They imply (although they do not state specifically) that this phenomenon is unique to the vertical scar technique, and the adjustment must be made in patients undergoing this method of reduction. I believe that this is a universal phenomenon in breast reduction, and the heavier the breast (ie, the larger the weight of reduction), the more the nipple "moves up" after surgery. The stretched skin "relaxes" and the nipple ends up at a higher level after surgery. I use this information in 2 ways: First of all, the larger the breast, the lower I place the nipple marking. Even more important, I adjust the initial marking position of the nipple to different heights when performing reduction in patients with significant breast asymmetry. I have not tried to quantify how much lower to place the nipple in a heavier breast, but I usually have been able to achieve symmetry within an acceptable range. (Maybe my patients with significant preoperative asymmetry are willing to accept slight asymmetry postoperatively.)

**R. L. Ruberg, MD**

**Lowering the Postoperative High-Riding Nipple**
Colwell AS, May JW Jr, Slavin SA (Harvard Med School, Boston, MA)
*Plast Reconstr Surg* 120:596-599, 2007

*Background.*—When reshaping the female breast, placement of a nipple too high creates an unnatural appearance that is invariably unacceptable to the patient. The surgical options to revise nipple placement are limited and create new scars. A repair technique employing infraclavicular tissue expansion was used to increase the absolute notch-to-nipple distance without leaving more superior scars.

*Methods.*—Three patients with abnormally high nipple placement during breast reduction or augmentation/mastopexy procedures participated. None were amenable to simple skin or scar excision or revision to revise the nipple placement. The technique using infraclavicular tissue expansion began with a periareolar incision or use of the existing reduction mammaplasty scar. The subcutaneous space just below the clavicle was tunneled into with crescent-shaped or round expanders. These were filled and maintained for several weeks until the desired nipple position was achieved or until the patient became unable to tolerate further expansion. The expander was then removed and lower pole revision surgery was performed.

*Results.*—No complications developed in the patients treated with infraclavicular tissue expansion. The notch-to-nipple distance was increased from 2 cm to 6 cm.

*Conclusions.*—The infraclavicular tissue expansion technique uses existing scars or periareolar incisions, producing no new scarring in the superior areas of the breast. When nipple elevation is severe, this technique offers a novel approach to the problem (Fig 2).

▶ I selected this article because I have always been frustrated by the problem of trying to lower a nipple that ends up too high after surgery (on someone else's

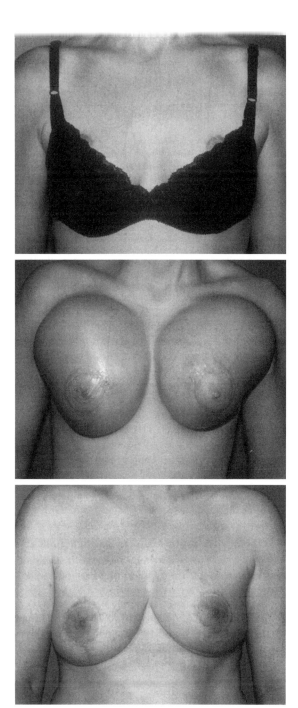

FIGURE 2.—Preoperative (*above*), expansion (*center*), and postoperative (*below*) photographs from one patient with high-riding nipples after reduction mammaplasty. This 37-year-old woman desired correction of superiorly malpositioned nipples that were visible when she was wearing a bra. Round expanders were filled to 1000 ml to lower the nipples 6 cm on each side. We do not routinely use implants with expander removal; however, small textured implants were placed in this patient to help maintain the inferior nipple position. Postoperative photographs are shown from her 1-year follow-up. (Reprinted from Colwell AS, May JW Jr, Slavin SA. Lowering the postoperative high-riding nipple. *Plast Reconstr Surg.* 2007;120:596-599, with permission from the American Society of Plastic Surgeons.)

patient, of course!). This technique should have been obvious to me, but it wasn't. The authors were able to use their method successfully in 3 patients. My only complaint about the report is the quality of the patient photos. The only preoperative picture shows the patient wearing a bra. The nipples are partly visible, but a photo without the bra would have allowed a better visualization of the magnitude of the change produced by the technique. Obviously, the best way to deal with this problem is to prevent it.

**R. L. Ruberg, MD**

---

**The Interlocking Gore-Tex Suture for Control of Areolar Diameter and Shape**
Hammond DC, Khuthaila DK, Kim J (Ctr for Breast and Body Contouring, Grand Rapids, MI)
*Plast Reconstr Surg* 119:804-809, 2007

---

*Background.*—During periareolar surgery one challenge is to avoid excessively widening and distorting the areola. A combination approach using Gore-Tex suture material and an interlocking purse-string technique was described.

*Technique.*—The "new" areolar diameter ranges from 44 to 52 mm. The area is marked while the areola is under maximal tension using a multidiameter circular areolar template. The areolar incision is made, the outer periareolar mark is incised and the skin between is deepithelialized. Five mm from the outer periareolar incision, the dermis is divided circumferentially, creating a dermal shelf to serve as a scaffold for placing the Gore-Tex suture to support periareolar closure. The breast flaps are circumferentially undermined around the periareolar opening for 1 to 2 cm directly beneath the dermis. The breast flaps can then be gathered in using the purse-string suture without bunching up or remaining attached to other tissues. Esthetic procedures can then be undertaken. Once the final breast size and shape are set, the periareolar defect is closed. The discrepancy between the larger outer incision circumference and the smaller inner incision is handled by evenly gathering the tissues together in a modified interlocking purse-string suture. The areola and outer periareolar incision are marked with eight evenly spaced points. Suturing commences at the most medial point of the periareolar defect, beginning in the deep tissues, passing through the dermal shelf, and emerging in the superficial tissues. The needle makes evenly spaced passes through the dermal shelf, following the cardinal points, and intersperses small "bites" of areolar dermis. This interlocks the outer purse-string closure with the inner areolar incision and creates a distinctive wagon wheel configuration.

*Conclusions.*—A stable areolar size and shape are achieved by locking the outer periareolar incision into the inner incision. The Gore-Tex suture possesses excellent qualities for this application, permitting easy control of the areolar diameter.

▶ The article provides photo documentation of several cases in which a previously unsuccessful periareolar closure is significantly improved using this technique. I would agree with the authors that it must be the combination of both unique technique and very specialized suture that allows control of the recalcitrant periareolar scar. Of course, the surgeon and the patient must be prepared to accept the presence of a permanent suture just beneath the periphery of the areola.

**R. L. Ruberg, MD**

**Bicompartmental breast lipostructuring**
Zocchi ML, Zuliani F (C. S. M. Institute for Aesthetic Plastic Surgery, Torino, Italy)
*Aesthet Plast Surg* 32:313-328, 2008

The techniques of additive mastoplasty described over the years require the use of alloplastic materials (silicon), which often are poorly tolerated by the body and need access paths that could leave visible, unaesthetic residual scars. Furthermore, the controversy over silicone gel-filled breast implants, which in the early 1990s restricted their clinical use for primary cosmetic breast augmentation, still raises concerns in some patients. The authors therefore felt encouraged to search for alternatives to breast implants and reconsider fat transfer. In fact, for almost a century, autologous adipose tissue has been used safely and with success in many other surgical fields for the correction of volumetric soft tissue defects. Its natural, soft consistency, the absence of rejection, and the versatility of use in many surgical techniques have always made autologous adipose tissue an ideal filling material. In the past, the authors used this technique, as originally described by Fournier (intraparenchymal, en bloc injection), for 41 patients. However, disappointed by a very high rate of complications and the almost complete reabsorption of the grafted fat, they quit using the procedure. An extensive literature review indicated that the complications observed were related only to technical errors and to the anatomic site of harvesting and implantation. The authors therefore developed a new method incorporating recent contributions in functional anatomy and fat transfer. Fat is harvested in a rigorously closed system, minimally manipulated, and reimplanted strictly in two planes only: into the retroglandular and prefascial space and into the superficial subcutaneous plane of the upper pole of the breast (bicompartmental grafting). Any intraparenchymal placement is carefully avoided. Since 1998, 181 patients (300 breasts) have undergone this procedure. Grafted fat volume has ranged from 160 to 685 ml (average, 325 ml) per breast. Complications have been minimal and temporary. All patients have been carefully monitored with preoperative and serial postoperative mammograms and ultrasonograms. This strict follow-up assessment allowed the authors to clarify the controversial aspect of microcalcifications, the main point of criticism for this procedure over the years. Microcalcifications can occur in response to any trauma or surgery of the breast, but are very different in appearance and location. Thus, they can be discriminated easily from those appearing in the context of a neoplastic focus. Probably the most important point is that the fat survival ranged from 40% to 70% at 1 year. The volume is maintained because when the authors transplant living fat tissue, they also transfer a consistent amount of adult mesenchymal stem cells that spontaneously differentiate into preadipocytes and then into adipocytes, compensating for the partial loss of mature adipocytes reabsorbed through time. This theory has been well demonstrated via advanced research performed by the authors and by many other prominent medical institutes worldwide. The findings show that adipose tissue has the same potential for growth of adult mesenchymal totipotential stem cells of bone marrow and can eventually be differentiated easily by the use of specific growing factors and according to the needs and applications in other cellular lines (osteogenic, chondrogenic, myogenic, epithelial). In summary, the authors wish to highlight a formerly controversial procedure that, thanks to recent technical and clinical progress, has become a safe and viable alternative to the use of alloplastic materials for breast augmentation for all cases in which additive mastoplasty with implants is either unsuitable or unacceptable by the patient herself. However this method

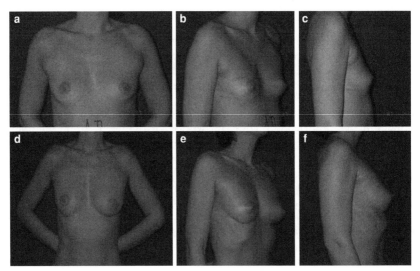

FIGURE 12.—(a-c) Preoperative views of a 30-year-old woman with a severe breast hypotrophy. (d-f) Postoperative views 2 years after a bicompartmental breast lipostructuring procedure that reimplanted 290 ml of adipose tissue in each breast. (Reprinted from Zocchi ML, Zuliani F. Bicompartmental breast lipostructuring. *Aesthet Plast Surg.* 2008;32:313-328, with permission from Springer Science+Business Media.)

cannot be considered yet as a complete substitute for augmentation with implants because the degree of augmentation and projection still is limited (Fig 12).

▶ This is an important article about an important subject. Fat grafting for breast enlargement is growing in popularity, but not without some controversy. The authors present a series of patients in whom fat grafting has been done successfully using their own technique. There appears to be no question that they are able to achieve modest breast enlargement without the use of implants. However, in today's world of breast augmentation, modest enlargement would not be enough for many patients. Among the many controversies are the following: The authors claim that centrifugation of the fat is not needed—other authors claim that it is. The authors use external breast skin expansion and claim that this modality improves graft take. Others achieve a high degree of graft take without external expansion.[1] Finally, the authors claim that their success is based upon the "bicompartmental" placement of fat. No fat is placed into the breast itself. There is no evidence given for the value of this approach. Nevertheless, one must conclude that fat grafting for breast enlargement works.

**R. L. Ruberg, MD**

*Reference*

1. Coleman SR, Saboeiro. Fat grafting to the breast revisited: safety and efficacy. *Plast Reconstr Surg.* 2007;119:775-785.

---

**Liposuction Breast Reduction: A Prospective Trial in African American Women**
Moskovitz MJ, Baxt SA, Jain AK, et al (Image Plastic Surgery, Paramus, NJ; Cosmedical Plastic Surgery, Paramus, NJ, New Jersey Inst of Technology, Paramus; et al)
*Plast Reconstr Surg* 119:718-726, 2007

---

*Background.*—Recently published case reports and outcome studies support the use of liposuction alone as an effective technique for ameliorating symptoms of breast hypertrophy. This study is the first prospective trial to examine the effectiveness of liposuction breast reduction as a primary modality of breast reduction. In addition, this study examines the role that liposuction breast reduction can play in the treatment of African American women, given the known scarring difficulties that darker skinned patients can encounter with traditional breast reduction surgery.

*Methods.*—Twenty African American women were recruited through newspaper and Internet advertisements. Patients aged 20 to 60 years were serially accepted to the study. Patients with a chief complaint of breast ptosis were excluded. No other exclusion criteria were used. Previously validated questionnaire instruments were used preoperatively and postoperatively to measure breast-related symptoms, general patient health perception, bodily pain, and self-esteem. Comorbid conditions, demographics, financial status, prior treatments, and smoking history were also documented.

*Results.*—Seventeen patients completed the preoperative and postoperative questionnaires. An average of 1075 cc of tissue was removed per breast during liposuction breast reduction surgery. Postoperative assessment showed a significant decrease in breast-related symptoms, a significant decrease in patient pain, and a significant improvement in overall patient health perception.

*Conclusions.*—Liposuction breast reduction is a useful breast reduction modality in the properly selected patient. African American women, who may traditionally forego breast reduction surgery because of scarring, are excellent candidates for this type of reduction procedure.

▶ The results shown by the authors, are impressive (see figure in the original article). Of greatest importance, is the fact that the authors were able to correlate their good aesthetic results with documented relief of symptoms. It is well established that conventional breast reduction techniques produce a high rate of symptom relief, but this is (I think) the first demonstration that liposuction alone can have the same benefit. One important question: Will insurance companies ever agree to cover this form of "non-surgical" breast reduction?

**R. L. Ruberg, MD**

---

**Large-Volume Reduction Mammaplasty: The Effect of Body Mass Index on Postoperative Complications**
Gamboa-Bobadilla GM, Killingsworth C (Med College of Georgia, Augusta; Univ of Alabama at Birmingham)
*Ann Plast Surg* 58:246-249, 2007

---

Eighty-six women underwent modified inferior pedicled reduction mammaplasty. All were grouped according to body mass index (BMI): 14 in the overweight group, 51 in the obese group, and 21 in the morbidly obese group. The mean ages were 34, 35, and 36, respectively, for the 3 groups and were not statistically different. The mean resection weight in the overweight group was 929 g, 1316 g for the obese group, and 1760 g for the morbidly obese group. Wound healing complications increased with BMI; the overweight, obese, and morbidly obese groups had 21%, 43%, and 71% of complications, respectively. The results were not statistically different. The rate of repeat operations increased proportionally with the BMI to 7%, 8%, and 19%, respectively. Postoperative BMI was measured in 30 patients. Fifty percent of this group had limited preoperative activity secondary to breast enlargement. The mean postoperative follow-up period was 43 months. Forty-seven percent of this group continued to have limited activity after breast reduction, with a mean BMI of 37.8 kg/m². The mean BMI of all women was 37.41 kg/m², with a total BMI change of −0.4 kg/m², suggesting that most women do not lose a significant amount of weight after breast reduction. There was no statistical difference in long-term BMI.

▶ The authors divided their patients into 3 groups (overweight, obese, and morbidly obese), looked at complication rates, and concluded that there was no statistically significant difference between the three groups. I think that one can take a different approach with the same data and come to a different conclusion. My reassessment of their data is as follows: Patients with a BMI less than 30 kg/m² had a 21% complication rate (3/14); patients with a BMI over 30 kg/m² had a 51% complication rate (37/72). I think the study just didn't have enough patients, or didn't organize the data effectively to demonstrate statistical significance (see Table in the original article). I would be very cautious with patients whose BMI is above 30, and I would be prepared to deal with complications in these patients.

**R. L. Ruberg, MD**

---

**The Impact of Breast Size on the Vertebral Column: A Radiologic Study**
Findikcioglu K, Findikcioglu F, Ozmen S, et al (Gazi Univ, Ankara, Turkey)
*Aesthetic Plast Surg* 31:23-27, 2007

---

*Background.*—Macromastia usually is associated with the physical and psychological symptoms reported, comprehensively, by many studies. Reduction mammoplasty seems to be the most reasonable solution for these symptoms, and many articles have reported improvement of these complaints after surgery. Some authors have postulated that the anatomic mechanisms of postural aberrations are heavy breasts and related pain symptoms. However, limited numbers of studies have tried to explain the effect of the heavy breasts on the vertebral column.

*Methods.*—This study enrolled 100 females in four groups according to their breast cup sizes (groups A, B, C, D). All four groups were compared with each other, statistically; using one-way analysis of variance (ANOVA) followed by a post hoc test according to the body mass index (BMI), as well as the thoracic kyphosis, lumbar lordosis, and sacral inclination angles.

*Results.*—The BMI was significantly higher in the D cup–sized breast group. There was a statistically significant difference between groups A and D, in terms of the thoracic kyphosis and the lumbar lordosis angles, and between groups B and D in terms of the lumbar lordosis angle. No statistically significant difference was detected between the groups, in terms of the sacral inclination angle.

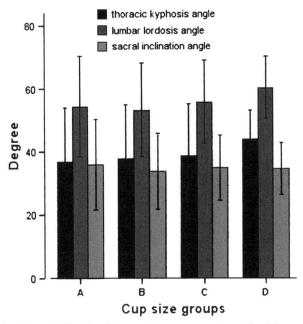

FIGURE 3.—The vertebral angles of the cup size groups are shown. The differences between the thoracic kyphosis angles of group A and D, and between the lumbar lordosis angles of group A and D as well as groups B and D are significant ($p < 0.05$, ANOVA). There is no significant difference between the sacral inclination angles of the groups ($p > 0.05$, ANOVA) (T above the bar depicts standard deviation). (Courtesy of Findikcioglu K, Findikcioglu F, Ozmen S, et al: The impact of breast size on the vertebral column: a radiologic study. *Aesthetic Plast Surg* 31:23-27, 2007. Reprinted with permission from Springer Science+Business Media, LLC.)

*Conclusion.*—Breast size seems to be an important factor that affects posture, especially the thoracic kyphosis and lumbar lordosis angles (Fig 3).

▶ The authors present the first step, in another form of assessment, of the benefit of breast reduction. They are able to show the effect of increasing breast size in producing deformity of the vertebral column (see figure). Reassessing these measurements after reduction mammaplasty would be most interesting. Would improvement in symptoms (which we know is almost always achieved) correlate with measureable changes in the vertebral column?

**R. L. Ruberg, MD**

## Lactational Performance after Breast Reduction with Different Pedicles

Cruz NI, Korchin L (Univ of Puerto Rico, San Juan)
*Plast Reconstr Surg* 120:35-40, 2007

*Background.*—Uncertainty still exists as to whether one type of pedicle is superior to another in preserving the breastfeeding potential of young women who need breast reduction surgery.

*Methods.*—The lactational performance of women who had breast reduction surgery with different pedicle types was compared with that of women of child-bearing age with macromastia but no prior breast surgery. Of those who had reduction mammaplasty, 48 had superior, 59 had medial, and 57 had inferior full-thickness dermoglandular pedicles. A total of 151 women with macromastia, but without prior breast surgery, comprised the control group. All women completed a questionnaire on breastfeeding success. Successful breastfeeding was defined as breastfeeding for 2 weeks or more. The women were also classified as having breastfed exclusively or with supplementation.

*Results.*—Of the women in the control group who attempted to breastfeed, 62 percent were successful. Breastfeeding success rates for patients who had breast reduction surgery were 62 percent for superior pedicle, 65 percent for medial pedicle, and 64 percent for inferior pedicle. No significant difference ($p > 0.05$) was found between groups. Thirty-four percent of the control group supplemented breastfeeding, and no significant difference was found between the control group and the patients who had breast reduction surgery with superior (38 percent), medial (38 percent), and inferior (35 percent) pedicles. Loss of nipple sensation was 2 percent for all pedicle types.

*Conclusion.*—The lactational performance of women who had breast reduction surgery using superior, medial, or inferior full-thickness pedicles was not significantly different from that of women with macromastia but no breast surgery.

▶ There are 2 important pieces of information in this article. First of all, only about two thirds of patients with macromastia were successful in breast feeding, which is not close to the 100% that most of us would have guessed. Second, no matter what one would guess the influence of pedicle location to be on successful lactation, it didn't matter what technique was used—the same percentage of patients were able to breast feed. We must throw out the guesses and go with the data. We can conclude that there is NO reduction in the ability to breast feed successfully after reduction mammaplasty.

**R. L. Ruberg, MD**

**One-Stage Mastopexy with Breast Augmentation: A Review of 321 Patients**
Stevens WG, Freeman ME, Stoker DA, et al (Univ of Southern California Los Angeles, CA)
*Plast Reconstr Surg* 120:1674-1679, 2007

*Background.*—One-stage mastopexy with breast augmentation is an increasingly popular procedure among patients. In the past 9 years, there has been a 506 percent increase in mastopexy procedures alone. Although some recommend a staged mastopexy and breast augmentation, there are currently no large studies evaluating the safety and efficacy of a one-stage procedure.

*Methods.*—A retrospective chart review was conducted of 321 consecutive patients who underwent one-stage mastopexy and breast augmentation. Data collected included the following: patient characteristics, implant information, operative technique, and postoperative results Complication and revision rates were calculated to evaluate the safety and efficacy of the one-stage procedure.

*Results.*—No severe complications were recorded over an average of 40 months' follow-up. The most common complication was deflation of a saline implant (3.7 percent), followed by poor scarring (2.5 percent), recurrent ptosis (2.2 percent), and areola asymmetry (2.2 percent). Forty-seven patients (14.6 percent) underwent some form of revision surgery following the one-stage procedure. Thirty-five (10.9 percent) of these were for an implant-related issue, whereas 12 patients (3.7 percent) underwent a tissue-related revision. This 10.9 percent implant-related revision rate is less than a previously documented 13.2 percent 3-year reoperation rate for breast augmentation alone. The authors' 3.7 percent tissue-related revision rate also compares favorably to an 8.6 percent revision surgery rate in patients who underwent mastopexy alone.

*Conclusions.*—Although it has been stated that the risks of a one-stage procedure are more than additive, the results of our review suggest otherwise. Although a revision rate of 14.6 percent is significant, it is far from the 100 percent reoperation rate required for a staged procedure.

▶ The increasing popularity of mastopexy combined with breast augmentation makes this information particularly useful to all plastic surgeons. The authors correctly identify this as a technically challenging operation with a high incidence of complications. The patient must be extensively counseled with regard to both the nature and the likelihood of complications requiring surgical revision. This article gives the surgeon sufficient information to counsel patients adequately and accurately. As long as the patient is willing to proceed in face of the significant complication rate, then combining these 2 procedures into 1 operative experience is reasonable and appropriate. More information from this review would be beneficial to the surgeon, but it has not provided 1 major piece of information about the relationship of the technique used for mastopexy to the incidence of complications. Anecdotal information suggests that "donut" mastopexy techniques may have the highest incidence of complications. The answers to this and other questions may be available from future studies.

**R. L. Ruberg, MD**

# Augmentation and Silicone

### A Retrospective Analysis of 3,000 Primary Aesthetic Breast Augmentations: Postoperative Complications and Associated Factors
Araco A, Gravante G, Araco F, et al (Crown House Hosp, Birmingham, England; Univ of Tor Vergata in Rome, Italy; et al)
*Aesthetic Plast Surg* 31:532-539, 2007

*Background.*—A large retrospective analysis was performed on a homogeneous group of patients undergoing primary aesthetic breast augmentations to define complication rates and find associated factors.

*Methods.*—Data were collected from the personal databases of two different surgeons working at the Crown House Hospital, Oldbury, Birmingham, United Kingdom. The period considered was January 1996 to December 2001. All patients who received primary breast augmentation with or without associated mastopexy for cosmetic purposes were recorded.

*Results.*—A total of 3,002 women were included in the study. Hematomas were present in 46 patients (1.5%), infections in 33 patients (1.1%), breast asymmetries in 23 patients (0.8%), rippling in 21 patients (0.7%), and capsular contractures in 14 patients (0.5%). The multivariate analysis found that implant placement and the technique used for pocket creation were variables associated with complications ($p < 0.05$). Capsular contractures carried a progressive cumulative risk and, in our series, appeared 5 years after surgery. No association was found between contractures and hematomas or infections.

*Conclusions.*—The overall incidence of complications in our series was relatively high (4.6%). Surgical placement of prostheses and the technique used for pocket creation were associated with complications. However, few patients required reoperation (1.6%), and the overall satisfaction rate was acceptable (visual analog score, 7) (Table 2).

▶ There is a wealth of information in this study. Some of this information is not translatable to practice in the United States because the implants used by these surgeons in the United Kingdom are not likely the same as those used in the United States. But the remainder of the information (eg, technique for pocket creation, position of the implant, use of drains) is probably applicable in the United States. Unfortunately, one cannot use this study to conclude that one approach is clearly better than all the others, because of the balance of advantage and disadvantage for some of the parameters, which were measured. For example, the submuscular/dual-plane approach resulted in an elevated rate of hematoma, but a reduced rate of breast asymmetry. Another disadvantage of the article is that it is simply a retrospective, rather than a prospective,

TABLE 2.—Results of Univariate and Multivariate Analysis For Each Complication Analyzed

| Complication | Univariate Analysis | Multivariate Analysis |
|---|---|---|
| Hematomas | Mentor prostheses (protect.) | — |
| | PIP | — |
| | Submuscular/dual-plane approach | Submuscular/dual-plane approach |
| | Manual pocket creation | Manual pocket creation |
| Infections | Antibiotics for pocket washing (protect.) | — |
| | Mentor prostheses (protect.) | — |
| | Drains | — |
| Breast asymmetry | Submuscular/dual-plane approach (protect.) | Submuscular/dual-plane approach (protect.) |
| | Mentor prostheses (protect.) | — |
| | PIP prostheses | — |
| Rippling | Subglandular approach | Subglandular approach |
| | PIP prostheses | — |
| Capsular contractions | Manual pocket creation | — |
| | Drains | — |

(Reprinted from Araco A, Gravante G, Araco F, et al. A retrospective analysis of 3,000 primary aesthetic breast augmentations: postoperative complications and associated factors. *Aesthetic Plast Surg.* 2007;31:532-539, with permission from the Springer Science+Business Media.)

randomized study. Nevertheless, individual surgeons should be able to find much information, which will be useful for their own practices.

**R. L. Ruberg, MD**

## Advantages and Outcomes in Subfascial Breast Augmentation: A Two-Year Review of Experience

Siclovan HR, Jomah JA (Med Art Clinics, Riyadh, Saudi Arabia)
*Aesthet Plast Surg* 32:426-431, 2008

*Background.*—One of the most popular surgical cosmetic procedures, breast augmentation, has enjoyed large acceptance in the last few decades. One of the most important factors in the dynamics established between the implants and the soft tissues after breast augmentation is the pocket plane. Surgeons have been seeking the proper plane into which the implant might be placed. The subglandular approach resulted in implant edge visibility and was thought to result in a higher incidence of fibrous capsular contractures. Despite the advantage of concealing the implant edges using the subpectoral approach, implant displacement occurred with contraction of the pectoralis muscle. The use of the retrofascial plane seems to yield the benefits of both planes without the deficits.

*Methods.*—Since 2006, 45 patients with hypomastia have undergone subfascial breast augmentation using anatomical contour profile gel cohesive III textured implants.

*Results.*—Pleasing long-term results have been obtained by using subfascial breast augmentation, with maintenance of a natural breast shape and a smooth transition between the soft tissue and implant in the upper pole. There were no capsular contractures and no complaints regarding displacement of the implants with contraction of the pectoralis major muscle.

*Conclusions.*—The subfascial breast augmentation technique offers improved long-term aesthetic results because the dynamics between the implant and soft tissues have been optimized. This technique is extremely

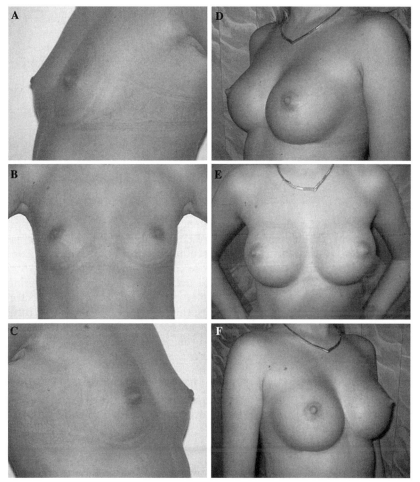

FIGURE 2.—(A, B) Preoperative frontal and oblique views of a 22-year-old patient. (D, E) Postoperative views after breast augmentation with 225-cc anatomical implants medium height, high profile in the subfascial plane; result after six months. (Reprinted from Siclovan HR, Jomah JA. Advantages and outcomes in subfascial breast augmentation: a two-year review of experience. *Aesthet Plast Surg.* 2008;32:426-431, with permission from the Springer+Business Media.)

versatile and may also be used in patients requiring removal and replacement of breast implants (Fig 2).

▶ The results demonstrated in this article are quite good. We do not see photos of a large number of patients, but those that are shown demonstrate a breast contour, which to me looks quite natural (ie, not "augmented"). I am not sure whether this shape is the result of the type of implant or the subfascial placement—probably, it is a combination of these 2 factors. Am I ready to adopt this technique? Probably not. The authors indicate that this approach requires more careful (and I assume more time-consuming) dissection, and entails more bleeding than either subglandular or submuscular techniques. If patients were desirous of avoiding the "augmented," rounder look of the breasts after surgery, then application of this technique might be reasonable. In my experience most patients are actually happy with the "augmented" appearance, so for me the extra effort required for this approach is not needed. Other surgeons may disagree, and in such a circumstance this subfascial approach could be a good choice.

**R. L. Ruberg, MD**

---

**Complete Submuscular Breast Augmentation: 650 Cases Managed Using an Alternative Surgical Technique**
Hendricks H (KÖ-Klinik GmbH, Düsseldorf, Germany)
*Aesthetic Plast Surg* 31:147-153, 2007

---

*Background.*—An alternative complete submuscular surgical technique for primary breast augmentation is presented. Since 1998, the author has refined the procedure for total submuscular placement of textured silicone gel implants, with good results for more than 650 patients.

*Methods.*—The submuscular plane is accessed via a semicircular periareolar incision. Round or anatomic implants are placed beneath the pectoralis major and external oblique muscles, the rectus sheath, and the serratus anterior muscle fascia, which together create a contiguous structure that completely separates the implant from the breast tissue.

*Results.*—High-riding implants were the main complication in early cases, through creation of an insufficiently large submuscular pocket. Only a very low incidence of Baker II capsular fibrosis was observed, and there were no Baker III or IV capsular contracture revisions. There were no cases of infection or "bottoming out." Areolar scarring was well concealed, and rippling and implant distortion were virtually nonexistent. Even in thin women, the implant edge was scarcely visible or palpable. Patient satisfaction levels were very high, with the majority viewing the implants as their own tissue, in terms of natural feel and appearance.

*Conclusions.*—The advantages of the described surgical method are several-fold, particularly for lean patients. It offers a promising alternative to subglandular and partial submuscular implant placement and to other

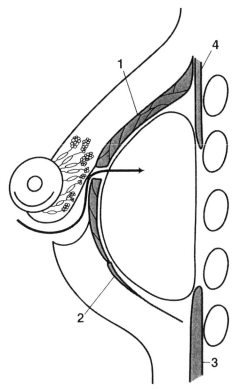

FIGURE 1.—A 3- to 4-cm inferior circumareolar incision is made, avoiding damage to the retroareolar gland and sensory tissue. Blunt transection of the pectoralis major muscle is at the level of the third intercostal space. [1] pectoralis major muscle, [2] rectus sheath with external oblique muscle, [3] rectus abdominis muscle, [4] pectoralis minor muscle. (Reprinted from Hendricks H, Complete submuscular breast augmentation: 650 cases managed using an alternative surgical technique. *Aesthetic Plast Surg.* 31:147-153, 2007. with permission from Springer Science+Business Media, LLC.)

total submuscular techniques for primary breast augmentation. Furthermore, it provides a solution for tuberous and ptotic breasts, coupled with mastopexy, as required, and good results have been achieved with correctional surgery for subglandular capsular contracture, bottoming out, and rippling (Fig 1).

▶ The question remains as to whether this technique should be done. I think that the technique (Fig 1) does hide the implant more effectively than any other approach, but the extra time needed to learn the procedure, and then to perform the operation, may not be worth the effort. The article shows that complete submuscular breast augmentation can be done with a high success rate. For those who see this method as desirable; this article provides useful guidance and detail.

**R. L. Ruberg, MD**

## Subpectoral Breast Augmentation Through the Abdominoplasty Incision

Rinker B, Jack JM (Univ of Kentucky, Lexington)
*Ann Plast Surg* 58:241-245, 2007

---

Abdominoplasty and breast augmentation are often performed together, and subglandular augmentation through the abdominoplasty incision has been previously described. Nine cases of subpectoral breast augmentation and abdominoplasty performed through a single low transverse abdominal incision were performed between 2002 and 2005. The selection criteria included women who were healthy, nonsmokers, without true breast ptosis or breast deformity requiring additional shaping. The subpectoral space was accessed and the pectoralis major origins were mobilized under direct vision, and the implant pocket was shaped with the aid of a breast sizer and breast dissector. The mean follow-up was 22 months. The surgical goals were realized in all cases, with no asymmetry or implant-related complications. The standard abdominoplasty incision provides ample exposure for the creation of a subpectoral pocket and precise placement of implants. The procedure should be considered in patients who wish abdominal recontouring and breast augmentation and have minimal ptosis (Fig 3).

▶ This approach to placement of breast implants has been described before. The value of this study is the number of patients (9) and the lack of breast complications in this series. Therefore, one can conclude not only that this procedure can be done, but also that it can be done safely in most patients. The limits of this approach have not been tested because the authors will carefully control the extent of the abdominal dissection, will not do associated liposuction, and will not do the procedure on smokers. All these steps are taken to

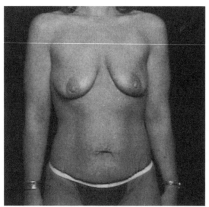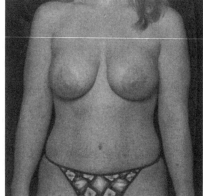

FIGURE 3.—Above Left, Thirty year old woman, preoperative, frontal view. Above, Right Thirty-one months following transabdominoplasty subpectoral breast augmentation with 390-mL implants, front view. (Reprinted from Rinker B, Jack JM Subpectoral breast augmentation through the abdominoplasty incision. *Ann Plast Surg.* 2007;58:241–245, with permission from the Lippincott Williams & Wilkins.)

ensure that the additional dissection at the top of the abdomen does not compromise the blood supply to the abdominal skin, which is essentially a large flap. I think these steps are wise.

**R. L. Ruberg, MD**

**Relative Implant Volume and Sensibility Alterations After Breast Augmentation**
Pitanguy I, Vaena M, Radwanski HN, et al (Pontifical Catholic Univ of Rio de Janeiro, Brazil; Rua Dona. Mariana, Rio de Janeiro, Brazil)
*Aesthetic Plast Surg* 31:238-243, 2007

*Background.*—Recent studies have provided diverging results regarding the factors that may affect sensibility after primary breast augmentation. Implant volume is believed to be an important factor, but the relation of implant size to breast volume has not been adequately addressed. In addition, the literature shows that a conflict exists when the periareolar and inframammary approaches are compared. This study aimed to refine the volumetric analysis comparing the implant and final breast size as well as the intrinsic association of these two factors with postoperative sensory alteration of the breast.

*Methods.*—A prospective study investigated patients who underwent aesthetic breast augmentation between June 2004 and October 2005 (i.e., a 16-month period) at the Ivo Pitanguy Institute. The sensibility in nine regions of the breast was tested before and after surgery using Semmes-Weinstein monofilaments. Breast sizers were used to compare the pre- and postoperative breast volumes. Statistical analysis of the data took into consideration the relative volume of the implant, the surgical approach, the presence of minor complications, the breast-feeding history, and the subjective evaluation of sensory changes in the patients.

*Results.*—A total of 37 patients who underwent breast augmentation were examined preoperatively. The relative volume of the implant was found to be associated with sensibility alterations. No difference was found between the periareolar and inframammary incision approaches. Other factors such as previous breast-feeding, minor complications, and subjective alterations were not associated with sensory alterations.

*Conclusions.*—The study findings suggest that larger implants and smaller breasts show an increased association with postoperative sensory alterations of the breast. Plastic surgeons and their patients should be aware of this possibility. Implant volume should be considered together with breast size to avoid sensory complications, and this is summarized in the concept of relative volume.

▶ I think that this is really useful information, but only if the patient is really concerned about breast sensibility after augmentation mammaplasty. This study (albeit in a small group of patients) clearly suggests that the patient with small breasts who wants to be big is very likely to have permanently reduced sensation postoperatively. There is a current trend that recommends that the implant size is best determined by the patient's chest size. In general, this would probably mean that a small person shouldn't receive a large implant. But if the patient tells her surgeon that size is more important than sensibility, then a large implant can be justified (with appropriate informed consent).

**R. L. Ruberg, MD**

---

### Silicone Gel Implants in Breast Augmentation and Reconstruction
Gampper TJ, Khoury H, Gottlieb W, et al (Dept of Plastic Surgery, Charlottesville, VA; Univ of Virginia Health System, Charlottesville, VA; Private Practice, Mclean, VA)
*Ann Plast Surg* 59:581-590, 2007

---

Silicone gel implants have been widely used for breast augmentation and reconstruction since the 1960s. Several alterations to both elastomer shell and filler gel have been made over the years to improve their ability to replicate the natural breast and to decrease the incidence of capsular contracture. The latter is a pathologic process involving the periprosthetic tissues formed in response to the presence of the implant. When severe, capsular contracture may cause firmness, distortion, and pain. In response to many claims of implant-related connective tissue disease, the US Food and Drug Administration placed a moratorium in 1992 on silicone gel breast implants for cosmetic purposes. Despite a preponderance of scientific data to their safety, silicone gel implants are presently available in the United States only as part of limited clinical trials. They continue to be used in Europe and other parts of the world.

▶ This article is selected not because it provides any new information (it does not), but because it is an up-to-date, comprehensive review of all relevant information related to silicone gel breast implants. All plastic surgeons who use these valuable devices should be familiar with the history, the complications, and the advantages and disadvantages of these implants. A major value of this article is the extensive bibliography that the authors supply. The surgeon, therefore, has access not only to a brief description of each complication and each described use of gel implants, but also has the ability to easily find a more comprehensive description through the appropriate references in the medical literature. The authors make no judgments about the different types of implants, different placement sites, etc; they just provide access to information that the individual surgeon can use to make an intelligent personal choice.

**R. L. Ruberg, MD**

### Soft cohesive silicone gel breast prostheses: a comparative prospective study of aesthetic results versus lower cohesivity silicone gel prostheses

Panettiere P, Marchetti L, Accorsi D (Università degli Studi di Bologna, Italy; Poliambulatorio Privato Dr Pietro Panettiere, Bologna, Italy)
*J Plast Reconstr Aesthetic Surg* 60:482-489, 2007

The flexibility of lower cohesivity silicone prostheses is the main reason for wrinkling, rippling and evidence of implant edges. The soft cohesive silicone implants promise to minimize such effects with minimal softness reduction.

Forty consecutive patients received soft cohesive prostheses (INAMED® Style 110 ST™) and were studied prospectively. A historical group, made up by the 40 consecutive patients who received lower cohesivity silicone implants (INAMED® Style 110™) in the immediately preceding months, was used as a control.

Wrinkling, prosthetic edge perceptibility and capsular contracture degree were assessed six months after surgery. The tissue coverage thickness was measured using ultrasonography. The patients were then asked to evaluate the breast softness by means of an anonymous questionnaire, where they also expressed their overall satisfaction by means of the five-steps linear analogical scales.

The wrinkling prevalence was 9.2% in the soft cohesive group vs. 55% in the lower cohesivity one ($p < 0.01$). The edge perceptibility was 14% in the soft cohesive group vs. 22% in the lower cohesivity one (no statistical significance). The coverage tissue thickness was not found to be significantly related to the wrinkling prevalence or to the edge perceptibility. The capsular contracture rate was almost identical in the two groups (Baker II: 2.6% vs. 2.7%, no Baker III or IV). A higher stiffness was noted in the soft cohesive group (average score: 4.2 vs. 4.4 in the control

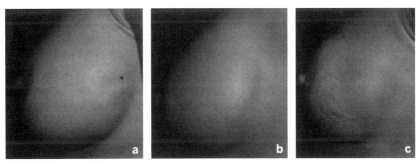

FIGURE 1.—Visible defects of prostheses in the LC group. (a) Visible rippling; (b) visible border; and (c) visible rippling and visible border. No visible defect was found in the SC group. (Reprinted with permission from Panettiere P, Marchetti L, Accorsi D. Soft cohesive silicone gel breast prostheses: a comparative prospective study of aesthetic results versus lower cohesivity silicone gel prostheses. *J Plast Reconstr Aesthetic Surg.* 2007;60:482-489. Copyright 2007, British Association of Plastic, Reconstructive and Aesthetic Surgeons.)

group, $p < 0.05$), but the overall satisfaction degree was higher for soft cohesive implants (average score: 4.5 vs. 3.8, $p < 0.01$).

The soft cohesive prostheses offered better overall results than the lower cohesivity silicone prostheses, even if a longer term follow-up should be advised. The soft cohesive prostheses showed a higher firmness, but this seemed not to have any influence on the overall satisfaction degree (Fig 1).

▶ Although this is a retrospective rather than a prospective study, the conclusions seem to be logical and useful. In essence, when the 2 types of implants are available for general use (which they are not at the time of this writing), the surgeon and the patient can make a choice based on the most important quality desired by the patient. If minimal wrinkling and implant edge palpability are the most desired characteristics, then the more cohesive implant will fulfill these objectives. On the other hand, if a more natural breast-like feel is desired, then the less cohesive implant produces this result. The authors conclude that the more cohesive implant gives better overall results, but this conclusion is only valid in the context of the patient's desires as described previously.

**R. L. Ruberg, MD**

---

**Filling of Adjustable Breast Implants Beyond the Manufacturer's Recommended Fill Volume**
Becker H, Carlisle H, Kay J (Boca Raton, FL)
*Aesthet Plast Surg* 32:432-441, 2008

---

*Background.*—Adjustable breast implants are widely used for both reconstructive and cosmetic breast surgery. They provide unique postoperative versatility and allow for more effective management of numerous conditions that would otherwise require surgical intervention. Findings have shown that in a clinical setting, it often is necessary to overexpand saline implants beyond the manufacturer's recommended fill volumes for positive results and optimal patient satisfaction. The authors investigated their breast-augmentation patients, comparing implants expanded beyond the manufacturer's fill volume with implants that remained within the recommended parameters.

*Methods.*—A total of 138 patients (270 implants) undergoing breast augmentation mammoplasty with Smooth Round Spectrum implants were evaluated postoperatively. To determine the effects of overexpansion, the incidence of leakage was assessed as well as the possibility of increased firmness. Patients completed a satisfaction questionnaire.

*Results.*—The findings showed no evidence of increased leakage with implants expanded beyond recommended fill volumes, and 97% of the patients reported a perfect score for satisfaction ratings. Of the 270 implants evaluated in the study, only 7 were given a less than perfect score.

*Conclusions.*—By exceeding the recommended fill volume, the authors were able to use the implant to its maximal potential, with increased patient satisfaction. The authors were able to correct problems and avoid complications that could not have been resolved without deviating from the manufacturer's recommended fill volumes. Nonvalidated restrictions on fill volumes severely limit the efficacy of adjustable implants.

▶ This is a valuable article because it confirms that adjustable implants can be safely filled in vivo to volumes greater than those recommended by the manufacturers. However, the question still remains as to whether implants should be filled to these volumes. I think overfilling makes sense in selected situations, but not necessarily those that are documented in this study. These authors intentionally overfilled a large number of implants used for augmentation mammaplasty. Their rationale principally was that patients decided some time after their surgery was completed that they wanted larger implants. The authors left filling valves in place so that they could accomplish this adjustment at a later date. My own philosophy is that the surgeon should comply with manufacturer's recommendations as often as possible. In the short time of this study, no implants ruptured. But over time, some of these implants will rupture. Will the intentionally overfilled implants still be covered by the manufacturer's warranty? I don't think so. Therefore, my solution to the problem of postoperative change in volume desired by the patient is to do a better job preoperatively of implant selection. Different surgeons have different ways of doing this. In my practice I reserve intentional overfilling to those reconstructive cases (particularly cases of breast asymmetry) in which my preoperative judgment of the necessary final volume was incorrect (ie, too little). In this circumstance, overfilling can be justified in lieu of another operation to place a larger implant.

**R. L. Ruberg, MD**

---

**Excess Mortality From Suicide and Other External Causes of Death Among Women With Cosmetic Breast Implants**
Lipworth L, Nyren O, Ye W, et al (Internatl Epidemiology Inst, Rockville, MD; Vanderbilt Univ, Nashville, TN; Karolinska Institutet, Stockholm)
*Ann Plast Surg* 59:119-123, 2007

---

An increased rate of suicide among women with cosmetic breast implants has been consistently reported in the epidemiologic literature. We extended by 8 years the follow-up of our earlier mortality study of a nationwide cohort of 3527 Swedish women with cosmetic breast implants to examine in greater detail suicide and other causes of death. The number of deaths observed among these women was compared with the number expected among the age- and calendar-period-matched general female population of Sweden. Women with breast implants were followed for over 65,000 person-years, with a mean follow-up of 18.7 years (range, 0.1–37.8 years). Overall, 175 deaths occurred among women with breast implants versus 133.4 expected (standardized mortality ratio (SMR) = 1.3; 95% confidence interval [CI], 1.1–1.5).

Among women with implants, we observed statistically significant 3-fold excesses of suicide (SMR, 3.0; 95% CI, 1.9–4.5) and deaths from alcohol or drug dependence (SMR, 3.1; 95% CI, 1.0–7.3), as well as an excess of deaths from accidents and injuries consistent with substance abuse or dependence. The increased risk of suicide was not apparent until 10 years after implantation. Deaths from cancer overall were close to expectation (SMR, 1.1; 95% CI, 0.8–1.4). Women with cosmetic implants had elevated SMRs for lung cancer and chronic respiratory disease. There was no excess of breast cancer mortality. The excess of deaths from suicides, drug and alcohol abuse and dependence, and other related causes suggests significant underlying psychiatric morbidity among these women. Thus, screening for pre-implant psychiatric morbidity and post-implant monitoring among women seeking cosmetic breast implants may be warranted (Table 2).

▶ Several previous articles have purported to show an increase in suicide in women after cosmetic breast augmentation. I think most plastic surgeons were hopeful that additional studies, with more patients follow up, would negate this disturbing finding. Unfortunately, the opposite is true: This study extended by 8 years the follow-up of patients in a previous study published of Swedish women, and the same conclusion is reached. In addition, several

TABLE 2.—Standardized Mortality Ratios (SMRs) and 95% Confidence Intervals (CIs) for Total Mortality and Selected Causes of Death Among 3527 Swedish Women With Cosmetic Breast Implants

| Cause of Death | Observed | Expected | SMR | 95% CI |
|---|---|---|---|---|
| All causes | 175 | 133.4 | 1.3 | 1.1–1.5 |
| All cancers | 63 | 57.5 | 1.1 | 0.8–1.4 |
| Digestive tract | 7 | 14.0 | 0.5 | 0.2–1.0 |
| Lung | 21 | 8.2 | 2.6 | 1.6–3.9 |
| Breast | 11 | 14.0 | 0.8 | 0.4–1.4 |
| Female genital | 9 | 9.2 | 1.0 | 0.4–1.9 |
| Cervix | 4 | 2.0 | 2.0 | 0.5–5.0 |
| Brain and nervous system | 2 | 2.7 | 0.7 | 0.1–2.6 |
| Hematopoietic | 10 | 4.4 | 2.3 | 1.1–4.2 |
| Circulatory system diseases | 31 | 29.5 | 1.0 | 0.7–1.5 |
| Ischemic heart disease | 8 | 13.5 | 0.6 | 0.3–1.2 |
| Cerebrovascular disease | 13 | 8.4 | 1.6 | 0.8–2.7 |
| Respiratory diseases* | 12 | 5.6 | 2.1 | 1.1–3.7 |
| Mental disorders† | 7 | 2.7 | 2.6 | 1.1–5.4 |
| Liver cirrhosis | 3 | 1.8 | 1.6 | 0.3–4.8 |
| Injuries and accidents‡ | 13 | 8.6 | 1.5 | 0.9–2.6 |
| Suicide | 24 | 8.0 | 3.0 | 1.9–4.5 |

*Includes pneumonia, bronchitis, emphysema, and asthma.
†Includes alcohol dependence (n = 3), drug dependence (n = 2), anorexia nervosa (n = 1), and dementia (n = 1).
‡Includes drug poisoning of unknown intent (n = 6), house fires (n = 2), exposure to cold (n = 1), hit by car (n = 1), car accident without collision by another car (n = 1), residential fall of unknown intent (n = 1), and occupant death in car accident (n = 1).
(Reprinted from Lipworth L, Nyren O, Ye W, et al. Excess mortality from suicide and other external causes of death among women with cosmetic breast implants. *Ann Plast Surg.* 2007;59:119-123, with permission from the Lippincott Williams & Wilkins.)

other causes of death that one could consider to be psychiatric diagnoses were also found to be increased. No one is suggesting that the implants cause the deaths; instead, the information is intended as a warning for physicians to screen these patients more carefully both before and after breast augmentation.

**R. L. Ruberg, MD**

---

**Cancer Risk among Los Angeles Women with Cosmetic Breast Implants**
Deapen DM, Hirsch EM, Brody GS (Univ of Southern California, Los Angeles)
*Plast Reconstr Surg* 119:1987-1992, 2007

---

*Background.*—As the first generation of women who received cosmetic breast implants ages, questions remain about cancer risk. This study is an update of the Los Angeles Augmentation Mammaplasty Study and examines cancer risk among women with long-term exposure to breast implants.

*Methods.*—The authors conducted a record linkage cohort study of patients with cosmetic breast implants by abstracting from records of the private practices of 35 board-certified plastic surgeons in Los Angeles County, California. They included 3139 Caucasian women who received cosmetic breast implants between 1953 and 1980. Spanish-surnamed women, nonresidents of Los Angeles County, and patients with prior subcutaneous mastectomy or breast cancer were excluded. Cancer outcomes through 1994 were ascertained through record linkage with the Los Angeles County Cancer Surveillance Program.

*Results.*—With a mean follow-up period of 15.5 years, 43 cases of breast cancer were observed, compared with 62.6 expected, based on Los Angeles County population-based incidence rates (standardized incidence ratio, 0.69; 95% CI, 0.50 to 0.93). Significant increases were observed for cancer of the lung and bronchus (standardized incidence ratio, 2.14; 95% CI, 1.42 to 3.09) and vulvar cancer (standardized incidence ratio, 3.47; 95% CI, 1.39 to 7.16).

*Conclusions.*—The breast cancer results of this study are consistent with the previous reports of the Los Angeles study as well as with several other long-term cohort studies. Lung cancer has previously been found to be increased in this cohort and also in some, but not most, other studies. The increased risk of vulva cancer has previously been observed in this cohort and just one other (Table 2).

▶ This article is another in the ongoing series of critical studies of breast implant patients that these authors have published. The essential conclusion, namely, that implants do not result in increased risk of breast cancer is maintained in every one of these reports, beginning with the first published in 1986. The other findings, including increased risk of lung and vulvar cancer, have been reported in other studies as well. These malignancies may reflect

TABLE 2.—Numbers of Observed and Expected Cancers, Standardized Incidence Ratios, and 95% Confidence Limits by Cancer Site, Los Angeles Augmentation Mammaplasty Study, 1972 to 1994*

| Cancer | No. Observed | No. Expected | SIR | 95% CI |
|---|---|---|---|---|
| Lund and bronchus | 28 | 13.1 | 2.14 | 1.42–3.09 |
| Endometrium | 9 | 9.2 | 0.98 | 0.45–1.86 |
| Ovary | 6 | 6.7 | 0.89 | 0.33–1.94 |
| Vulva | 7 | 2.0 | 3.47 | 1.39–7.16 |
| Invasive | 2 | 0.4 | 4.40 | 0.48–15.89 |
| In situ | 5 | 1.6 | 3.20 | 1.03–7.47 |
| Melanoma | 7 | 8.4 | 0.83 | 0.33–1.71 |
| Non-Hodgkin's lymphoma | 5 | 3.9 | 1.29 | 0.42–3.01 |
| Cervix | 6 | 5.3 | 1.13 | 0.41–2.46 |
| Rectum | 5 | 2.7 | 1.86 | 0.60–4.33 |
| Thyroid | 4 | 4.6 | 0.87 | 0.24–2.23 |
| Colon | 3 | 6.4 | 0.47 | 0.09–1.38 |
| Brain | 2 | 1.7 | 1.16 | 0.13–4.19 |
| Stomach | 2 | 1.1 | 1.90 | 0.21–6.87 |
| Pancreas | 2 | 1.6 | 1.22 | 0.13–4.41 |
| Anus | 2 | 0.4 | 4.44 | 0.49–16.03 |
| Sarcoma | 3 | 2.7 | 1.11 | 0.22–3.25 |

SIR, standardized incidence ratio.
**"Expected cancers" refers to invasive cancers only, unless otherwise specified. With regard to cancer site, one case was observed for each of the following: chronic lymphoid leukemia, carcinoid, mixed tumor of the genitalia, kidney cancer, meningioma, multiple myeloma, pituitary cancer, retroperitoneum/peritoneum cancer, and epithelial cancer of unknown primary site.

(Reprinted from Deapen DM, Hirsch EM, Brody GS. Cancer risk among Los Angeles women with cosmetic breast implants. *Plast Reconstr Surg.* 2007;119:1987-1992, with permission from the American Society of Plastic Surgeons.)

differences in social and behavioral characteristics of patients with implants compared with the normal population.

**R. L. Ruberg, MD**

# Cancer and Reconstruction

## Aesthetic Outcomes in Breast Conservation Therapy
Wang HT, Barone CM, Steigelman MB, et al (Univ of Texas Health Science Ctr at San Antanio, TX)
*Aesthet Surg J* 28:165-170, 2008

*Background.*—Since the National Surgical Adjuvant Breast and Bowel Project B06 (NSABP-B06) trial demonstrated equivalent survival outcomes between patients with breast cancer undergoing modified radical mastectomy versus lumpectomy and radiation, an increasing number of patients are seeking breast conservation therapy. Traditionally, only patients who have undergone total mastectomy have been referred for reconstruction.

*Objective.*—The purpose of the study was to determine the number of dissatisfied patients treated with breast conservation therapy who have suboptimal cosmesis and should be referred for reconstruction.

*Methods.*—After obtaining approval from the Institutional Review Board and patient consent, patients identified as more than 1 year post-treatment from breast conservation therapy (1999–2004) were interviewed and photographed. Data were gathered by use of a questionnaire that included patient aesthetic score, patient satisfaction, and change in body image. Photographs were shown to a surgical oncologist, a general surgeon, and a plastic surgeon for a physician aesthetic score.

*Results.*—Thirteen of 46 patients (28.3%) were dissatisfied with their cosmetic result. Women who were dissatisfied with their cosmetic result were more likely to have a negative change in their body image when compared with patients who were satisfied with their cosmetic result (46.2 % vs 6.1%, *P* =.02). Additionally, dissatisfied patients were more likely to rate their cosmetic result as poor (15.4 % vs 0%, *P* =.007) and were more likely to consider reconstruction (46.2% vs 9.1%, *P* =.01) when compared with satisfied patients. Risk factors to predict dissatisfaction in our patient population included age younger than 52 years and the resection of tumor from the upper inner quadrant.

*Conclusions.*—Twenty-eight percent of patients in this study were dissatisfied with their cosmetic result. Furthermore, a large portion of these patients would consider reconstruction if it were offered. Although this study only identified a few broad risk factors for suboptimal cosmetic outcome, it confirms our hypothesis that many patients who have undergone breast conservation therapy should be referred for plastic surgery consultation.

▶ There is a question that survival after breast conservation therapy (BCT) for breast cancer is equivalent to that achieved after mastectomy. I presume that its popularity is in part due to the perception of many physicians and patients that it is a less risky and less radical form of therapy and that the cosmetic results are better than after mastectomy. Unfortunately, data to support these 2 hypotheses are lacking. Anecdotal retrospective studies of patients selected by convenience—those still available and willing to participate—tend to limit the validity of the conclusions, even those that might be deemed reliable by virtue of significance through statistical analysis. The present study looks at a group of patients representing less than 30% of the possible study population and fails to assure us that the patients not studied are similar or different in a wide variety of parameters than those studied. It is also of interest that some 80% of the patients with BCT in the reported patients were happy with their choice of BCT, yet 35% were dissatisfied with the cosmetic outcome of that choice. Of the 13 patients dissatisfied with the cosmetic result, less than half would opt for reconstruction. This seeming dichotomy requires further study. It is important to consider the preponderance of a single ethnocentric group in the population studied, and the cultural implications this potentially has for generalizing the results of this study. To reliably and validly assess the issue of comparability of patient satisfaction with the BCT procedure and cosmetic outcomes, it would be useful to have a prospectively conducted and reported study by a multicenter surgical collaborative with at least arms—those with BCT alone and those with BCT followed by reconstruction.

**S. H. Miller, MD, MPH**

---

**Periareolar Skin-Sparing Mastectomy and Latissimus Dorsi Flap with Biodimensional Expander Implant Reconstruction: Surgical Planning, Outcome, and Complications**
Munhoz AM, Aldrighi C, Montag E, et al (Univ of São Paulo, Brazil)
*Plast Reconstr Surg* 119:1637-1649, 2007

---

*Background.*—Although use of the latissimus dorsi myocutaneous flap associated with the Biodimensional anatomical expander implant system (McGhan 150) is a reliable technique, little information has been available regarding clinical outcome following periareolar skin-sparing mastectomy reconstruction. The purpose of this study was to analyze the feasibility of the technique, surgical planning, and its outcome following skin-sparing mastectomy.

*Methods.*—Thirty-two patients underwent immediate unilateral latissimus dorsi myocutaneous flap/Biodimensional anatomical expander implant system breast reconstruction. Mean follow-up was 18 months. The technique was indicated in patients with small- or moderate-volume breasts with or without ptosis, in whom the use of abdominal flaps was precluded. Flap and donor-site complications were evaluated. Information on anesthetic results and patient satisfaction was collected.

*Results.*—Seventy-two percent had tumors measuring 2 cm or less (T1), and 78 percent were stage 0 and I according to American Joint Committee on Cancer criteria. Breast skin complications occurred in 9.4 percent. Two patients presented small breast skin necrosis, and in one patient, a wound dehiscence was observed. Donor-site complications, all represented by seroma, occurred in 12.5 percent. The cosmetic result was considered good or very good in 84.4 percent, and the majority of patients were either very satisfied or satisfied. No local recurrences were observed. All complications, except two, were treated by conservative means.

*Conclusions.*—The latissimus dorsi myocutaneous flap/Biodimensional anatomical expander implant system is a simple and reliable technique for periareolar skin-sparing mastectomy reconstruction. Success depends on patient selection, coordinated planning with the oncologic surgeon, and careful intraoperative and postoperative management.

▶ This is a nice study with good results, documenting the outcome of breast reconstruction with a latissimus dorsi flap, combined with the use of a biodimensional anatomic expander implant. For the most part, the authors confined their study and report to patients with small tumors and patients with small to moderate-volume breasts.

The skin paddle of the latissimus flap seems to be small, and one wonders if a larger skin paddle might have been used to fill more of the defect with blood bearing tissue (de-epithelialized extra skin), rather than relying heavily on the implant.

A complication rate comparable to other studies is reported, but the contribution of radiation to these and the aesthetic outcome was not performed, due to small sample sizes. Follow-up is short, and it would be very interesting to see these patients studied again, in the future, along with an assessment of whether the rate of complications increases or decreases with time, as well as whether patients with complications were more or less satisfied than those without complications.

**S. H. Miller, MD, MPH**

---

**Breast Cancer Recurrence Following Prosthetic, Postmastectomy Reconstruction: Incidence, Detection, and Treatment**
McCarthy CM, Pusic AL, Sclafani L, et al (Memorial Sloan-Kettering Cancer Center, NY)
*Plast Reconstr Surg* 121:381-388, 2008

---

*Background.*—The purpose of this study was to evaluate the influence of prosthetic reconstruction on the incidence, detection, and management of locoregional recurrence following mastectomy for invasive breast cancer.

*Methods.*—A matched retrospective cohort study was performed. Only patients with invasive breast cancer who had 2 years or more of follow-up and/or patients who had recurrence within 2 years of their primary cancer were included.

*Results.*—In total, 618 patients who underwent mastectomy for invasive breast cancer from 1995 until 1999 were evaluated. Three hundred nine patients who had immediate, tissue expander/implant reconstruction were matched to 309 women who underwent mastectomy alone on the basis of age ($\pm 5$ years) and breast cancer stage (I, II, or III). The incidence of locoregional recurrence following mastectomy was 6.8 percent in patients who had reconstruction and 8.1 percent in patients who had mastectomy alone (log rank $p = 0.6015$). Median time to detection of a locoregional recurrence was 2.3 years (range, 0.1 to 7.2 years) in the reconstructed cohort and 1.9 years (range, 0.1 to 8.8 years) in the nonreconstructed cohort ($p = 0.733$). Permanent implants were removed following infection in one patient and patient request in two.

*Conclusions.*—These results suggest that there is no difference in the incidence of locoregional recurrence in breast cancer patients who undergo immediate, tissue expander/implant reconstruction compared with those patients who do not have reconstruction. Prosthetic breast reconstruction does not appear to hinder detection of locoregional cancer recurrence. In the majority of patients, management of locoregional recurrence does not necessitate removal of a permanent prosthesis.

▶ We are now beginning to get better and more scientifically sound evidence that breast reconstruction, at least using prosthetic implants, does not increase the risk of recurrence, be it locoregional or distant. I presume that the category of distant recurrence, mentioned in this study, includes metastatic breast cancer in both cohorts. I am less convinced than the authors that estrogen receptor status and tumor size are not important variables. Their experience that detection of cancer recurrence is not hindered by the presence of prosthetic implants certainly mirrors mine. It would be of interest to repeat this study in patients undergoing autologous tissue reconstruction and compare the demographics and end points with matched patients reconstructed by prosthesis and those just undergoing mastectomy.

**S. H. Miller, MD, MPH**

**Prospective Analysis of Long-term Psychosocial Outcomes in Breast Reconstruction: Two-year Postoperative Results From the Michigan Breast Reconstruction Outcomes Study**
Atisha D, Alderman AK, Lowery JC, et al (Univ of Michigan Med Ctr, Ann Arbor, MI; Ann Arbor VA Health Care System, MI; et al)
*Ann Surg* 247:1019-1028, 2008

*Objective.*—To prospectively evaluate the psychosocial outcomes and body image of patients 2 years postmastectomy reconstruction using a multicenter, multisurgeon approach.

*Background.*—Although breast reconstruction has been shown to confer significant psychosocial benefits in breast cancer patients at year 1 postreconstruction, we considered the possibility that psychosocial outcomes may remain in a state of flux for years after surgery.

*Methods.*—Patients were recruited as part of the Michigan Breast Reconstruction Outcome Study, a 12 center, 23 surgeon prospective cohort study of mastectomy reconstruction patients. Two-sided paired sample *t* tests were used to compare change scores for the various psychosocial subscales. Multiple regression analysis was used to determine whether the magnitude of the change score varied by procedure type.

*Results.*—Preoperative and postoperative year 2 surveys were received from 173 patients; 116 with immediate and 57 with delayed reconstruction. For the immediate reconstruction cohort, significant improvements were observed in all psychosocial subscales except for body image. This occurred essentially independent of procedure type. In the cohort with delayed reconstruction, significant change scores were observed only in body image. Women with transverse rectus abdominis musculocutaneous flaps had significantly greater gains in body image scores ($P = 0.003$ and $P = 0.034$, respectively) when compared with expander/implants.

*Conclusions.*—General psychosocial benefits and body image gains continued to manifest at 2 years postmastectomy reconstruction. In addition, procedure type had a surprisingly limited effect on psychosocial well being. With outcomes evolving beyond year 1, these data support the need for additional longitudinal breast reconstruction outcome studies.

▶ This is a very important study because of its collaborative approach to addressing the questions posed and the use and timing of instruments designed to evaluate the end results. Although not a randomized controlled trial (RCT), the study does make use of multiple surgeons in multiple locations and thus the results are more likely generalizable than a study conducted in a single center or by a single surgeon. Of some concern is the low response rate between years 1 and 2 and the differences between the 2 groups suggesting that the nonresponders were doing less well than the responders. The authors did detect that those with immediate reconstruction had better outcomes at the 2-year mark than did those who underwent delayed reconstruction. Was the delayed reconstruction group homogenous in terms of when reconstruction occurred? Might there be some psychological and timing factors, all other things being equal, that would enable one to predict which patients might do better after delayed reconstruction?

**S. H. Miller, MD, MPH**

## Psychological Factors Predict Patient Satisfaction with Postmastectomy Breast Reconstruction

Roth RS, Lowery JC, Davis J, et al (Univ of Michigan Health System, Ann Arbor; Veterans Affairs Ctr for Practice Management and Outcomes Research, Ann Arbor, Mich)
*Plast Reconstr Surg* 119:2008-2015, 2007

*Background.*—This prospective study examined the contribution of psychological factors to the prediction of patient satisfaction with postmastectomy breast reconstruction surgery.

*Methods.*—Women presenting for breast reconstruction were administered presurgical psychological inventories. Measures of affective distress, depressive symptoms, anxiety, somatization, and somatic preoccupation were obtained from standardized inventories. At 1-year ($n = 295$) and 2-year ($n = 205$) follow-up, subjects completed ratings of their satisfaction with both the general and aesthetic results of surgery.

*Results.*—After controlling for sociodemographic variables and both surgical procedure type and timing, multiple linear regression analyses indicated that at 1-year follow-up preoperative measures of affective distress, depression, somatization, and somatic anxiety predicted less general satisfaction with surgical outcome, while presurgical levels of affective distress, depression, anxiety, somatization, and somatic anxiety predicted decreased aesthetic satisfaction. At 2-year follow-up, only preoperative affective distress retained a significant association with lowered general satisfaction with reconstructive surgery. In addition, at 2-year reassessment, aesthetic quality of surgical outcome was inversely related to all the presurgical psychological variables.

*Conclusions.*—Affective distress and somatic preoccupation negatively influence patient satisfaction with both aesthetic and general outcomes associated with postmastectomy breast reconstruction. Presurgical psychological screening and counseling of selected women, who are being considered for breast reconstruction, may be advisable to enhance patient satisfaction with reconstructive surgery.

▶ This is a very large, well-conducted study of several psychological factors, which may be associated with the outcomes of postmastectomy reconstruction. Findings that premastectomy reconstruction psychological symptoms, including depression, affective distress, somatic fears, and bodily complaints were generally associated with lower levels of postoperative satisfaction, reflect my experiences, in this regard.

Patient dissatisfaction after breast reconstruction is, unquestionably, a complex issue and requires more study, including an evaluation and comparison, pre- and postoperative, of body image and quality of life. Future studies should also be expanded to address the generalizability, or not, of the patient populations studied. Do patients in Michigan, Canada, and Pennsylvania react like those in New York or California? Nonetheless, the authors' suggestions to carefully evaluate the preoperative psychological status is valid.

**S. H. Miller, MD, MPH**

---

## A Retrospective Analysis of Patient Satisfaction with Immediate Postmastectomy Breast Reconstruction: Comparison of Three Common Procedures

Saulis AS, Mustoe TA, Fine NA (Northwestern Univ, Chicago)
*Plast Reconstr Surg* 119:1669-1676, 2007

---

*Background.*—The authors aimed to quantify overall patient satisfaction with three breast reconstruction techniques and identify factors that have influenced satisfaction.

*Methods.*—Two hundred sixty-eight questionnaires were mailed at least 6 months after immediate breast reconstruction to consecutive breast reconstruction patients over a 3-year period. A second questionnaire was sent out 9 months later to the tissue expander/implant group of patients.

*Results.*—The initial questionnaire demonstrated that overall satisfaction was significantly greater in the transverse rectus abdominis myocutaneous (TRAM) flap patients, as compared with the tissue expander/implant patients ($p < 0.05$). However, the number of patients willing to repeat the procedure and recommend their procedure to a friend was similar among all three reconstructive techniques. A significantly greater number of tissue expander/implant patients as compared with TRAM flap patients felt they had not received sufficient information to make an educated decision ($p < 0.05$). This finding correlated with the lower satisfaction rate among the tissue expander/implant patients. The second questionnaire sent only to the tissue expander/implant patients revealed that the majority felt uninformed about the final aesthetic outcome and the frequency and pain associated with the expansion process.

*Conclusions.*—All three groups may claim to be satisfied with their own personal choices. Many patients will continue to choose tissue expander/implant reconstruction in an effort to avoid scars and more extensive surgery. Being less satisfied is not wrong or bad, provided it is known. Tissue expander/implant patients should be thoroughly informed, in the preoperative setting, about the final aesthetic outcomes and the immediate perioperative expansion period, which may involve a considerable amount of patient commitment and discomfort in some women.

▶ The authors attempt to determine, by use of a retrospective analysis, patient satisfaction with immediate breast reconstruction, based on 3 different types of breast reconstructions: TRAM flap, latissimus dorsi flap with an implant, and expander/implant reconstruction.

Not surprisingly, patients with tissue expander/implant reconstructions appeared to be the least satisfied. This has certainly been reported by other authors.[1] The major finding in this study is that patient satisfaction correlates negatively with inadequate preoperative information, especially in the expander/implant group. Overall, the study suffers from its retrospective nature, problems with patient recall, timing of the questionnaire vis-à-vis the procedure, and perhaps, from knowing that the surgeons followed the same "script" and demeanor when informing their patients. I agree that patient satisfaction is vitally important when evaluating outcomes in plastic surgery. It is also true that patient satisfaction is multifactorial, and it behooves the plastic surgeon to identify those factors under his/her control and modify their patient interactions to lessen disappointment. Perhaps, it would be useful to have a trusted "agent," family member, or close friend, attend preoperative discussions with these patients and to show a spectrum of results, rather than the ideal result, for the procedures discussed.

**S. H. Miller, MD, MPH**

*Reference*

1. Alderman AD, Wilkins EG, Lowery JC, Kim M, Davis JA. Determination of pateint satisfaction in postmastectomy breast reconstruction. *Plast Reconstr Surg.* 2000;106:769-776.

### Outcome Following Removal of Infected Tissue Expanders in Breast Reconstruction: A 10-Year Experience
Halvorson EG, Disa JJ, Mehrara BJ, et al (Mem Sloan-Kettering Cancer Ctr)
*Ann Plast Surg* 59:131-136, 2007

Although several studies have analyzed risk factors for tissue expander removal prior to permanent implant placement in breast reconstruction, the outcome following explantation because of infection is unknown. From a prospectively maintained database covering a 10-year period, 39 such patients were identified. Twelve (30.8%) had prior radiotherapy. Nine patients (23%) underwent reexpansion, 3 (7.7%) had a latissimus dorsi flap and expander, and 1 (2.6%) received a free transverse rectus abdominis flap. Recurrent infection occurred in 1 reexpanded patient. Two patients developed late contractures. All other reconstructions were successful. Twenty-six patients (66.7%) did not undergo secondary reconstruction, most commonly due to a combination of patient preference, cancer progression, and radiotherapy. After removal of an infected expander, most patients who are interested and remain good candidates can still be reconstructed. Reexpansion was successful in patients without prior radiotherapy. Secondary reconstruction with autologous tissue is appropriate when there is a history of radiotherapy.

▶ Anyone who does breast reconstruction using tissue expanders with any degree of frequency has experienced postoperative infection requiring removal of the device. Many of these patients (as confirmed in this article) will give up (ie, they will decide that they just don't want any more surgery). In this series, most of the patients (26 of 39) decided to forgo additional reconstruction. In my personal experience, I find that most patients do want reconstruction. I have usually tried to replace the expander (because most of these patients elected tissue expansion because they wanted to avoid more complex procedures). I now have information from this study that confirms my impression: repeat expansion has a high likelihood of success.

**R. L. Ruberg, MD**

### Nipple Reconstruction: Evidence-Based Trials in the Plastic Surgical Literature
Momeni A, Becker A, Torio-Padron N, et al (Univ of Freiburg Med Ctr, Germany)
*Aesthet Plast Surg* 32:18-20, 2008

Although many technical descriptions of nipple reconstruction exist in the medical literature, insufficient evidence-based data are present about the outcome. This study aimed to identify randomized controlled trials (RCTs) and controlled clinical trials (CCTs) in the plastic surgical literature addressing nipple reconstruction, and to elucidate whether a hand search was superior to an extensive database search in retrieving all pertinent studies. The hand search included analysis of all "original articles" published in four of the leading plastic surgery journals, from January 1990 to December 2005, with subsequent identification of RCTs and CCTs. Additionally, a computerized search was conducted including the following databases: PubMed, Web of Science, and Evidence-Based Medicine Reviews. From a total of 10,476 published original articles in four plastic surgery journals over a 16-year period, only one RCT was identified that addressed nipple reconstruction. The database search, however, retrieved two trials: the RCT identified by hand search and one CCT. The impact of nipple reconstruction is well described in the literature. However, it is astonishing that the plastic surgical literature lacks evidence-based trials addressing this issue. Clearly, more evidence-based trials are necessary to ensure that recommendations for a particular technique are based on solid scientific data.

▶ Few, if any, doubt the veracity of the authors' primary conclusion that evidence-based literature to document the recommendations regarding surgical techniques, especially new plastic surgical techniques, is generally absent. Although nipple reconstruction is viewed as a minor procedure by most plastic surgeons, it is, nonetheless, a necessary, or at least desirable, finishing touch of most successful breast reconstructions. As any who have tried the "technique de jour" can attest, the long-term results rarely live up to the expectations, especially regarding long-term maintenance of nipple protrusion. I believe that the best basis for adopting a technique for nipple correction is reliance on series, which have adequate numbers of patients, followed for a minimum of 12 months.

**S. H. Miller, MD, MPH**

---

### The Influence of AlloDerm on Expander Dynamics and Complications in the Setting of Immediate Tissue Expander/Implant Reconstruction: A Matched-Cohort Study

Preminger BA, McCarthy CM, Hu QY, et al (New York Presbyterian Hosp-, Weill Cornell Med Ctr, NY; Mem Sloan-Kettering Cancer Ctr, NY)
*Ann Plast Surg* 60:510-513, 2008

---

AlloDerm (LifeCell, Branchburg, NJ) is gaining acceptance in tissue expander/implant (TE/I) breast reconstruction. Anecdotal evidence suggests its use limits postoperative musculoskeletal morbidity and allows injection of greater initial fill-volumes and rapid postoperative expansion. The objective of this study was to evaluate AlloDerm's impact on expansion rates in immediate TE/I reconstruction. A matched, retrospective cohort study was performed. Medical records of patients who underwent immediate TE/I reconstruction from 2004 to 2005 were reviewed. Two cohorts were identified: (1) underwent TE/I reconstruction with Allo-Derm, and (2) underwent standard TE/I reconstruction. Individuals were matched 1:1 on the basis of: expander size ($\pm$100 mL), history of irradiation, and indication for mastectomy. Cohorts were compared for intraoperative volume injected (mL), rate of postoperative expansion (mL/injection), number of expansions, and time to completion of expansion (days). Incidence of complications was evaluated. Pairwise comparisons were performed using the Wilcoxon sign rank test and McNemar test. Ninety immediate TE/I reconstructions were evaluated. Forty-five TE/I-AlloDerm reconstructions were matched to standard TE/I reconstructions. Intraoperatively, expanders in the AlloDerm and non-AlloDerm cohorts were filled to a mean volume of 223.8 and 201.1 mL ($P = 0.180$). Median number of expansions performed was 5 and 6 in the AlloDerm and non-AlloDerm cohorts ($P = 0.117$). There was no difference in the mean rate of postoperative tissue expansion (AlloDerm: 97 mL/injection versus non-AlloDerm: 95 mL/injection [$P = 0.907$]), nor in the incidence of complications ($P = 0.289$). Minor complications occurred in 13.1% of AlloDerm cases (cellulitis [n = 3], seroma [n = 3], hematoma [n = 1]. Although this study does not address AlloDerm's efficacy in decreasing morbidity or improving esthetic outcomes in TE/I reconstruction, it indicates that AlloDerm does not increase the rate of tissue expansion after immediate TE placement. It does not, however, appear to increase the risk of postoperative complications.

▶ By virtue of using a matched cohort study, the authors have begun to answer the question of whether AlloDerm is equivalent, in the rates of tissue expansion, to raising serratus muscle and rectus fascia to achieve total "muscle"—actually, autologus tissue coverage of tissue expanders. Apparently, in the authors' study, it appears to be. However, one must take into account that these patients were not randomized, that the observers and evaluators were not blinded as to which cohort had which treatment, and that at least some of the variables were dependent upon convenience (that is to say, when the patient and physician were available for filling of the tissue expander). It will be very worthwhile for the authors to present an outcome study of these same patients to evaluate aesthetic results, patient satisfaction contracture, effect of radiation, etc. Could AlloDerm be used to avoid raising the pectoralis muscle in reconstructed patients? Of course, should partial\total tissue coverage with AlloDerm be successful in reconstructive patients, might it also work for patients undergoing cosmetic augmentation?

**S. H. Miller, MD, MPH**

### The Cutaneous Arteries of the Anterior Abdominal Wall: A Three-Dimensional Study

Tregaskiss AP, Goodwin AN, Acland RD (Christine M. Kleinert Inst for Hand and Microsurgery, Louisville, KY; Univ of Louisville, KY)
*Plast Reconstr Surg* 120:442-450, 2007

*Background.*—Abdominal perforator flaps represent a natural progression in the quest to minimize abdominal wall morbidity. Their one disadvantage is the significant rate of vascular complications, to which they are subject in some series. The authors examined the vascular anatomy of the abdominal integument to determine why such complications occur and how they may be prevented.

*Methods.*—In 10 fresh cadavers, major arteries supplying the abdominal wall were injected with a lead-based contrast medium. The abdominal integument of each cadaver was imaged using a 16-slice spiral computed tomography scanner, to produce three-dimensional reconstructions of the arterial anatomy. Reconstructions were observed for orientation, course, and morphology of the major perforators within the abdominal integument.

*Results.*—Perforators of the deep inferior epigastric artery (DIEA) varied markedly in their orientation, course, and morphology among specimens. By contrast, perforators of the superior epigastric artery (SEA) were relatively consistent in their morphology and orientation. In eight of 10 specimens, SEA perforators with extensive anatomical "territories" orientated toward the umbilicus were present. These SEA perforators pierced the rectus sheath within 4 cm of the costal margin and were present bilaterally in seven of eight specimens.

*Conclusions.*—The unpredictable orientation and course of DIEA perforators indicate that the blood supply of abdominal perforator flaps, raised without clear knowledge of their unique vascular anatomy, may often be more random than axial. This may account for much of the ischemia-related morbidity observed with DIEA-based perforator flaps. Preservation of SEA perforators adjacent to the costal margin during abdominoplasty, will likely improve abdominal wall perfusion and reduce donor-site morbidity.

▶ This is an important cadaveric anatomic study of the tissues supplied by the deep inferior epigastric artery (DIEA) and the superior epigastric artery (SEA). Its importance lies in the large amount of variability of DIEA perforators. This may account for the unpredictability of DIEA-based flaps, as compared with SEA-based flaps.[1]

**S. H. Miller, MD, MPH**

*Reference*

1. Granzow JW, Levine JL, Chiu ES, Allen RJ. Breast reconstruction with the deep inferior epigastric perforator flap: history and update on current technique. *J Plast Reconstr Aesthetic Surg.* 2006;59:571-579.

### The Efficacy of Bilateral Lower Abdominal Free Flaps for Unilateral Breast Reconstruction

Beahm EK, Walton RL (Univ of Texas MD Anderson Cancer Ctr, Houston; Univ of Chicago Hospitals)
*Plast Reconstr Surg* 120:41-54, 2007

*Background.*—In large-breasted women, those with midline abdominal scars, or those with scant abdominal tissue, a unipedicled lower abdominal flap may be insufficient for breast reconstruction. In these circumstances, bipedicled flaps may best satisfy the reconstructive requirements, but outcomes with bilateral free flaps for unilateral breast reconstruction are generally lacking.

*Methods.*—A retrospective review of patients in whom two vascular pedicles/flaps were used to simultaneously reconstruct a single breast was used to assess operative outcomes.

*Results.*—Forty patients (80 flaps) for whom two free tissue transfers were used to simultaneously reconstruct a single breast were identified. The majority of patients had a native breast cup size of C or larger. The flaps used included the superficial inferior epigastric artery (SIEA) flap ($n = 29$; 36 percent), the transverse rectus abdominis musculocutaneous (TRAM) flap ($n = 9$; 11 percent), the muscle-sparing TRAM flap ($n = 15$; 19 percent), and the deep inferior epigastric perforator (DIEP) flap ($n = 27$; 34 percent). Flaps were paired in a variety of configurations, most commonly, using a muscle-sparing TRAM flap, in conjunction with a DIEP flap or an SIEA flap. Recipient vessels included a combination of the internal mammary and thoracodorsal vessels and the pedicles of combined flaps (turbocharged). There were no flap losses. Two flaps required reexploration for microsurgical anastomotic revision, and both were successfully salvaged. Isolated fat necrosis was encountered in only three of 80 flaps.

*Conclusions.*—This study suggests that bilateral, bipedicled, abdominal free flaps for unilateral breast reconstruction can be used safely, with a high degree of success. These combined flaps provide for enhanced vascular perfusion of the lower abdominal flap territory, allowing for harvest of larger volumes of tissue for reconstruction.

▶ This is a large series of patients in whom, for a variety of reasons, large breasts, midline abdominal scars, and paucity of donor abdominal skin, the authors reconstructed single breasts with bipedicle, bilateral abdominal free flaps in various combinations. They report no flap losses, but in light of the flexibility offered by using 2 flaps, each with its own blood supply, it was surprising to read that more than half of their patients required additional surgical contouring of the breast. Abdominal donor-site morbidity remains a problem, since it occurred in almost 8% of the patients, but only in those patients in whom the full width of the rectus was used. As the series progressed, the authors avoided using the full width of the rectus and began to use the more efficacious inlay mesh technique for facial repair, rather than simple overlay mesh repair. The algorithm, provided by the authors, is helpful.

The final caveat is that the operative time to complete the reconstructions is significant, averaging just under 9 hours, and requires an experienced team of microsurgeons. The latter accounts as much for the fact that they only had to take 2 patients back for vascular revisions and lost no flaps other than 2 with preoperative radiotherapy who developed native breast skin necrosis.

**S. H. Miller, MD, MPH**

---

**Full-Thickness Resection With Myocutaneous Flap Reconstruction for Locally Recurrent Breast Cancer**
Friedel G, Kuipers T, Dippon J, et al (Schillerhöhe Hosp at Robert Bosch Hosp, Gerlingen, Germany; Marienhosp, Stuttgart, Germany; Universität Stuttgart, Germany; et al)
*Ann Thorac Surg* 85:1894-1900, 2008

---

*Background.*—Despite available recommendations, therapeutic procedures of locally recurrent breast cancer are very different. This retrospective study presents the possibilities and results of complete, full-thickness chest wall resection.

*Methods.*—Between 1985 and 2006, 63 women (mean age, 58 years) with local recurrence of breast cancer invading the chest wall underwent chest wall resection with myocutaneous flap coverage and are included in this study. Adequate lung, cardiovascular, renal, and hepatic functions were additional eligibility requirements for inclusion. Preoperative known extrapulmonary metastases, pleural dissemination, and Eastern Cooperative Oncology Group (ECOG) status 3 or 4 were exclusion criteria. Survival rates were calculated by the Kaplan-Meier method. Univariable and multivariable Cox regression analysis was used for relative risk factors.

*Results.*—The median interval between operation for the primary tumor and of the local recurrence was 89 months, with median follow-up at 28 months. In the total collective, cumulative 5-, 10- and 15-year survival rates were 46%, 29%, and 22%, respectively, with a median survival of 56 months. R0 resection was associated with a 5-year survival of 50.4%. Prognostic factors were patient age at the time of the primary operation and tumor invasion of bony structures. Mortality was 1.6% and morbidity was 25%.

*Conclusions.*—Full-thickness chest wall resection of locally recurrent breast cancer performed by a team of thoracic and plastic surgeons provides the best survival rates, with low mortality and morbidity. An earlier application of this method may lead to further improvement of these results.

▶ This is an interesting study, not because it definitively provides evidence of increased longevity or reduction in morbidity of patients with local chest wall recurrence of breast cancer. It is important because it demonstrates that using the eligibility criteria they developed over a 20-year experience and a surgical team approach; it is possible to perform a potentially curative resection of full thickness chest wall recurrences of breast cancer. In the past, the presence of chest wall recurrence of breast cancer often signaled the beginning of the end for that patient. It has certainly been my experience that these patients, although few in any one surgeon's experience, when carefully chosen and cared for by an appropriate surgical and medical team can and do survive extended periods of time. Is it not time for a multicenter research approach to further refine the eligibility criteria, scope of surgery and reconstruction, and the proof that the recommendations of the author results in less mortality and morbidity than just treating these patients with palliative radiation or chemotherapy?

**S. H. Miller, MD, MPH**

# 7 Scars and Wound Healing

**Postoperative Radiation Protocol for Keloids and Hypertrophic Scars: Statistical Analysis of 370 Sites Followed for Over 18 Months**
Ogawa R, Miyashita T, Hyakusoku H, et al (Nippon Med School, Tokyo)
*Ann Plast Surg* 59:688-691, 2007

*Background.*—Before 2002, keloids and intractable hypertrophic scars were treated at our facility with postoperative irradiation of 15 Gy (the traditional protocol). Analysis of the therapeutic outcomes of patients treated with this protocol showed that the recurrence rates of keloids and intractable hypertrophic scars in the anterior chest wall, as well as the scapular and suprapubic regions, were statistically higher than at other sites, while the recurrence rates in earlobes were lower. Thus, we customized doses for various sites. This report describes our trial of postoperative radiation therapy.

*Methods.*—Between January 2002 and September 2004, 109 patients with 121 keloid and intractable hypertrophic scar sites were treated with surgical excision following the new protocol: electron-beam irradiation at total doses of 10, 15, or 20 Gy, depending on the site. The recurrence rates and toxicities were historically followed in 218 patients with 249 keloid and intractable hypertrophic scar sites treated with the old protocol of surgical removal followed by irradiation at 15 Gy (without variation by site). The minimal follow-up time was 18 months. Statistical analysis was performed using Fisher exact probability test.

*Results.*—Total recurrence rates were 29.3% before 2002 and 14.0% after 2003. The recurrence rate in the anterior chest wall was statistically reduced. Outcomes of earlobe did not differ between irradiation with 15 Gy or 10 Gy.

*Conclusions.*—Keloids and intractable hypertrophic scars should be treated with dose protocols customized by site. Our results suggest that keloid and intractable hypertrophic scar sites with a high risk of recurrence should be treated with 20 Gy in 4 fractions over 4 days and that earlobe should be treated with 10 Gy in 2 fractions over 2 days (Table 1 ).

▶ Like all of you, I struggle with the best way to treat keloids. Nothing seems to work completely. These authors describe their protocol with regionally stratified

TABLE 1.—Results of Our Study

| | Before 2002 (218 Patients) | | Since 2003 (109 Patients) | | |
| | Recurrence/Total | Rate (%) | Recurrence/Total | Rate (%) | P |
|---|---|---|---|---|---|
| Earlobe | 2/35** | 5.7 | 0/28* | 0.0 | 0.305 |
| Auricle excluding earlobe | 5/13** | 38.5 | 3/11** | 27.3 | 0.444 |
| Anterior chest wall | 32/82** | 39.0 | 5/35*** | 14.3 | 0.006 |
| Scapular region | 17/45** | 37.8 | 3/13*** | 23.1 | 0.262 |
| Suprapubic region | 8/22** | 36.4 | 2/10*** | 20.0 | 0.310 |
| Others | 9/52** | 17.3 | 4/24** | 16.7 | 0.611 |
| Grand total | 73/249 | 29.3 | 17/21 | 14.0 | 0.001 |

Cases followed over 18 month were selected. The therapeutic outcomes were analyzed statistically using Fisher exact probability test. A total of 218 patients with 249 regions (before 2002) and 109 patients with 121 regions (after 2003) were extracted for this study. The results suggest that keloid sites with a high risk of recurrence should be treated with 20 Gy/4 fractions/4 d. Moreover, earlobe keloids should be treated with 10 Gy/2 fractions/2 d. Total radiation dose: *10 Gy, **15 Gy, ***20 Gy.

(Reprinted from Ogawa R, Miyashita T, Hyakusoku H, et al. Postoperative radiation protocol for keloids and hypertrophic scars: statistical analysis of 370 sites followed for over 18 months. Ann Plast Surg. 2007;59:688-691, with permission from the Lippincott Williams & Wilkins.)

radiation dosing, showing significantly improved success. High-risk areas like the anterior chest are treated with 20 Gy with significant benefit compared with previous treatments. The complications are modest, although significant. Nevertheless, I will be sending this article to my radiation therapy colleagues. We may be increasing the dose we use for postoperative treatment and expect better results. You might consider the same.

**W. L. Garner, MD**

## The Results of Surgical Excision and Adjuvant Irradiation for Therapy-Resistant Keloids: A Prospective Clinical Outcome Study
van de Kar AL, Kreulen M, van Zuijlen PPM, et al (Academic Med Ctr, Amsterdam; Red Cross Hosp, Beverwijk, The Netherlands)
*Plast Reconstr Surg* 119:2248-2254, 2007

*Background.*—There is no consensus on the best way to treat keloids because adequate studies on this subject are sparse. Surgical excision, in combination with radiotherapy, is considered the most efficacious treatment available in severe keloids following the International Clinical Recommendations on Scar Management. Unfortunately, the recommendations are mainly based on retrospective studies that do not define recurrence.

*Methods.*—The authors evaluated the recurrence rate of therapy-resistant keloids treated with excision followed by radiotherapy (1200 Gy in three or four fractions). The minimum follow-up period was 12 months. The therapeutic outcome was judged as recurrence (elevation of the lesion not confined to the original wound area) or nonrecurrence. An evaluation of the outcome of the scars was obtained by using the Patient and Observer Scar Assessment Scale.

*Results.*—Twenty-one patients with 32 keloids were evaluated. The recurrence rate was 71.9 percent after a mean follow-up period of 19 months.

*Conclusions.*—This high recurrence rate suggests that radiotherapy might be less efficacious than suggested by other studies. On the basis of the authors' results, surgical excision, combined with radiotherapy, should be reserved as a last resort in the treatment of therapy-resistant keloids.

▶ Many articles have been written about the use of radiation therapy for control of keloids. This particular article is of value because of the strict criteria for defining success or failure, and the minimum of 12-month follow-up. The authors conclude that radiation therapy is really not a good choice for keloid treatment because it is successful in only about 30% of cases, and they recommend the use only as a last resort. I agree with this recommendation, but I have a different perspective on their data: I have *always* used radiation therapy only as a last resort, but now I can provide the patient with a better perspective regarding options for treatment. I will put a "positive spin" on the data and tell my patient that despite the failure of all previous treatments, this last resort can be successful in 30% of cases. I think many patients will accept this low chance of benefit in exchange for the possibility of eliminating a recalcitrant keloid.

**R. L. Ruberg, MD**

---

**The Efficacy of Topical Silicone Gel Elastomers in the Treatment of Hypertrophic Scars, Keloid Scars, and Post–Laser Exfoliation Erythema**
Chernoff WG, Cramer H, Su-Huang S (Chernoff Plastic Surgery and Laser Ctr, Santa Rosa, CA)
*Aesthetic Plast Surg* 31:495-500, 2007

---

*Background.*—Dermatix is a Food and Drug Administration (FDA)-registered substantial equivalent to silicone gel sheeting for the prevention and management of hypertrophic scars and keloids.

*Methods.*—A 90-day prospective study evaluated the efficacy of Dermatix, silicone gel sheeting, and a combination of these treatments in improving scars for 30 patients. Each patient had a bilateral scar that served as an untreated control. The outcome measures included profilometry analysis of scar topography before and after punch biopsies of the control and treated scars, symptoms associated with the scars, and patient evaluations of the ease of treatment.

*Results.*—The results showed better resolution and improvement of scars with Dermatix treatment or the combined use of Dermatix and silicone gel sheeting than with silicone gel sheeting alone. Wound erythema was reduced, and collagen architectural reorientation was demonstrated histologically. Patients rated Dermatix as easier to use than silicone gel sheeting. Both Dermatix and silicone gel sheeting reduced symptoms of itching, irritation, and skin maceration.

*Conclusion.*—The results of this study indicate that Dermatix is a useful treatment for the management of abnormal scarring.

▶ All of us treat scars nonoperatively. Although individual treatments have been proven beneficial, combination therapies have not been well studied. These authors studied the treatments they used as combination therapy; a silicone gel applied twice daily versus the use of silicone sheeting, both after laser treatment. The authors found significant that the gel caused improvement in the erythema and the scar elevation. The combination sounds like a simple and effective treatment, which I will now start to use. The success of the gel supports the idea that the charge of the silicone is what makes silicone sheeting work.

**W. L. Garner, MD**

---

## Scarring Occurs at a Critical Depth of Skin Injury: Precise Measurement in a Graduated Dermal Scratch in Human Volunteers

Dunkin CSJ, Pleat JM, Gillespie PH, et al (Stoke Mandeville Hosp, Aylesbury, England)
*Plast Reconstr Surg* 119:1722-1734, 2007

---

*Background.*—The association between scarring and the depth of dermal injury or burn is clinically recognized but not quantified. The authors tested the hypothesis that there is a critical depth beyond which a fibrous scar develops.

*Methods.*—A novel jig produced a wound that was deep dermal at one end and superficial dermal at the other. Pilot studies in cadaveric and ex vivo breast skin confirmed the depth of injury. Healthy volunteers had a standardized dermal wound made on the lateral aspect of the hip. Digital photography recorded the surface appearance of wound healing and scar development. High-frequency ultrasound demonstrated the depth of the healing wound and subsequent scar in vivo.

*Results.*—One hundred thirteen human subjects participated in the clinical study. Mean length of follow up was $28.6 \pm 13.2$ weeks. The deep dermal end of the wound healed with a visible scar and the superficial end had no visible residual mark after week 18. The initial length of injury was $51.3 \pm 0.6$ mm, which reduced to a scar of $34.9 \pm 1.0$ mm at 36 weeks (corresponding areas were $196.6 \pm 7.5$ mm$^2$ and $92.7 \pm 9.4$ mm$^2$). High-frequency ultrasound analysis showed a gradual reduction in scar thickness at the deep end and no detectable scar at the shallow end. The transition point between scar and no scar marked the threshold depth for scarring. This was calculated as $0.56 \pm 0.03$ mm, or 33.1 percent of normal hip skin thickness.

*Conclusions.*—The dermal scratch provides a well-tolerated, standardized, and reproducible wound model for investigating the healing response to dermal injury of different depths. There is a threshold depth of dermal injury at which scarring develops.

▶ It's good to have your clinical impressions verified by science. In this case, a study of scarring in normal people shows that deeper injuries cause more scarring. It is not surprising to any of us who have watched superficial lacerations heal perfectly and deeper ones heal with problems. The same applies to graft donor sites. For people doing wound-healing research, this is an excellent article to study methodologic advances. It provides proof that scarring is the result of a deeper dermal injury.

**W. L. Garner, MD**

---

**Shock Wave Therapy for Acute and Chronic Soft Tissue Wounds: a Feasibility Study**
Schaden W, Thiele R, Kölpl C, et al (AUVA-Trauma Ctr Meidling, Vienna; Zentrum für Extracorporale Stosswellentherapie, Berlin; Hadassah-Hebrew Univ, Mount Scopus, Jerusalem; et al)
*J Surg Res* 143:1-12, 2007

---

*Background.*—Nonhealing wounds are a major, functionally-limiting medical problem impairing quality of life for millions of people each year. Various studies report complete wound epithelialization of 48 to 56% over 30 to 65 d with different treatment modalities including ultrasound, topical rPDGF-BB, and composite acellular matrix. This is in contrast to comparison control patients treated with standard wound care, demonstrating complete epithelialization rates of 25 to 39%. Extracorporeal shock wave therapy (ESWT) may accelerate and improve wound repair. This study assesses the feasibility and safety of ESWT for acute and chronic soft-tissue wounds.

*Study Design.*—Two hundred and eight patients with complicated, nonhealing, acute and chronic soft-tissue wounds were prospectively enrolled onto this trial between August 2004 and June 2006. Treatment consisted of debridement, outpatient ESWT [100 to 1000 shocks/cm$^2$ at 0.1 mJ/mm$^2$, according to wound size, every 1 to 2 wk over mean three treatments], and moist dressings.

*Results.*—Thirty-two (15.4%) patients dropped out of the study following first ESWT and were analyzed on an intent-to-treat basis as incomplete healing. Of 208 patients enrolled, 156 (75%) had 100% wound epithelialization. During mean follow-up period of 44 d, there was no treatment-related toxicity, infection, or deterioration of any ESWT-treated wound. Intent-to-treat multivariate analysis identified age ($P = 0.01$), wound size $\leq 10$ cm$^2$ ($P = 0.01$; OR = 0.36; 95% CI, 0.16 to

0.80), and duration ≤1 mo ($P < 0.001$; OR = 0.25; 95% CI, 0.11 to 0.55) as independent predictors of complete healing.

*Conclusions.*—The ESWT strategy is feasible and well tolerated by patients with acute and chronic soft tissue wounds. Shock wave therapy is being evaluated in a Phase III trial for acute traumatic wounds.

▶ Frankly, I have no idea why this would work, but the authors are credible and contain some people who I know and trust completely. It seems like a simple enough intervention that might benefit many people with chronic wounds, but there are a couple of caveats. First, many interventions prove effective on patients with previously nonhealing wounds. This placebo effect from organized and attentive wound care makes conclusions of this kind of report uncertain. The next question is why would it work? There is significant evidence that wound debridement increases healing. Similarly, tissue damage with dermabrasion, laser resurfacing, or peels can stimulate healing in a positive way, so why not shock waves. Finally, a practical question: Can this be delivered with a hand held device? And if so, when are people going to be visiting my office to try to sell me one. Stay tuned folks; if this is real, I'm sure we'll hear more about it.

**W. L. Garner, MD**

---

### Vacuum Assisted Closure Device Improves the Take of Mesh Grafts in Chronic Leg Ulcer Patients
Körber A, Franckson T, Grabbe S, et al (Essen Univ School of Medicine, Germany)
*Dermatology* 216:250-256, 2008

---

*Background.*—Vacuum assisted closure (VAC) is established in the management of acute and chronic wounds. In recent years, few data have been published concerning VAC therapy after skin graft transplantation.

*Objectives.*—The aim of this study was to determine whether postoperative VAC helps assist closure of mesh grafts in chronic leg ulcer patients.

*Patients/Methods.*—We report a consecutive case series of 54 patients with chronic leg ulcers who received a total of 74 mesh grafts. A postoperative VAC therapy was performed in 28 mesh grafts, and 46 mesh grafts were treated with standard gauze therapy.

*Results.*—In the VAC group, 92.9% of grafts showed complete healing, compared to 67.4% in the control group without postoperative VAC therapy. Differential analysis revealed a negative correlation of the take rate in patients over 70 years of age or in patients suffering from diabetes mellitus or dermatoliposclerosis. Particularly patients with diabetes mellitus and of greater age exhibited improved take rates, both 100%, in the VAC group compared to 50 and 62%, respectively.

*Conclusion.*—The results of our retrospective study demonstrate for the first time the significant benefit of VAC therapy after skin grafting in chronic leg ulcer patients as evaluated in a clinical trial.

▶ The popularity of the vacuum-assisted closure (VAC) system for facilitating skin graft take has grown enormously. This article contributes more information about the value of this approach, but the conclusions of these authors cannot be judged as definitive because of some limitations in the study. I find that post-operative VAC therapy is particularly useful for skin grafts placed over irregular surfaces and places difficult to immobilize, such as the trunk. Traditional methods, such as "tie-over" dressings, do not always permit adequate immobilization and graft take may be problematic. On the other hand, grafts on the extremities are much easier to fix in place, and circumferential compression leads to a high level of graft "take." These authors claim that the VAC system results in a higher take than the traditional approach achieves. However, their study is a retrospective study, with the controls all being in a previously treated group. Several features of their "traditional" approach would differ from the methods that I use. First of all, when grafting a leg ulcer I almost always excise the bed of the ulcer before placing my graft (there is no indication that this was done in this study). Secondly, the dressings put on the grafts were not the same in the control and study groups. The control group had some form of silicone-impregnated dressing placed directly on the graft (something I never use), whereas the experimental group had the VAC sponge. We cannot be sure whether these factors influenced the take of the grafts. Also, there is no discussion of the relative cost of the 2 different treatment modalities, although one could make the case for a much more expensive form of dressing if it resulted in many fewer repeat grafting procedures. I do think that the VAC system has much to offer in facilitating skin graft take. This article gives us important information regarding a technique for grafting on the lower extremity—I just don't think that we should regard this as the final word on the superiority of this method.

**R. L. Ruberg, MD**

---

**New Continuous Negative-Pressure and Irrigation Treatment for Infected Wounds and Intractable Ulcers**
Kiyokawa K, Takahashi N, Rikimaru H, et al (Kurume Univ, Kurume City, Japan)
*Plast Reconstr Surg* 120:1257-1265, 2007

---

*Background.*—Continuous irrigation and the vacuum-assisted closure system are effective methods for the treatment of infected wounds and intractable ulcers. The objective of this study was to simultaneously use both of the above methods as a new approach for obtaining more satisfactory, accelerated wound healing.

*Methods.*—After debridement of the wound, indwelling irrigation and aspiration tubes are placed in the wounds that have been sutured closed.

With open wounds, a sponge with the same shape as the wound is placed directly onto the wound surface, and after the two tubes are inserted in the sponge, the wound is covered with film dressing to make the wound completely airtight. A bottle of physiologic saline solution is then attached to the irrigation tube, and a continuous aspirator (Mera Sacume) is attached to the aspiration tube. The bottle of physiologic saline solution is placed at the same height as the wound, and with a pressure gradient between the two of 0, continuous aspiration is applied.

*Results.*—All nine cases treated as closed air cavity wounds with this method healed after 2 to 3 weeks. In eight cases of open wound, recurrence of infection was observed in only one case.

*Conclusions.*—The two treatments of continuous irrigation and negative pressure were observed to have an additive and synergistic effect for earlier wound healing. Furthermore, the present method can dramatically reduce the number of dressing changes required, patient pain, psychological stress, and treatment cost.

▶ I've heard of people using this algorithm with the KCI VAC device. It doesn't make much sense to me because any irrigation would be rapidly aspirated from the wound and therefore only affect the surface of the wound. That process would have no predictable effect on the deeper wound tissues where infection, rather than wound surface colonization, is more important. As a result, I'm going to wait until someone studies this process in a more controlled setting. I'm not saying it doesn't work; I'm just saying it's one of those creative ideas that has yet been unproven.

**W. L. Garner, MD**

## Free Vascularized Fibula and Reconstruction of Long Bones in the Child–Our Evolution

Germain MA, Mascard E, Dubousset J, et al (Hôpital Saint Vincent de Paul, Paris)
*Microsurgery* 27:415-419, 2007

The aim is to show our evolution for reconstruction of long bones in the child with free vascularized fibula after tumoral resection. Between 1990 and 2004, 78 children were operated on for sarcoma of long bones and one girl with congenital pseudarthrosis. The main applications are illustrated: U-shaped fibular transplant, fibular epiphysis with growth plate and diaphysis transfer, fibular graft associated to massive allograft. Follow-up of the children was performed by clinical examination and standard X-ray. No post operative death occurred. Many benign complications for femoral reconstruction were observed. So our recent evolution is to use vascularized fibula associated with massive allograft; but resorption of allograft was observed 3 years later. Vascularized fibula for reconstruction of long bones is the ideal material. The result is definitive. The future for femur is perhaps vascularized fibula associated with osseous substitute.

▶ The techniques described in this series have essentially been reported previously. The value of the study is the compilation of multiple successful cases and the conclusions drawn by the authors. Even though there were multiple problems with the cases, the final result in virtually all instances was acceptable, although perhaps not ideal. The only problem with the study is that the authors' current recommended technique was not really tested; they simply determined that there were problems with resorption of allograft in the cases they were reporting, so the best technique was to use osseous substitute rather than allograft. I guess we have to wait for the next study to tell us whether osseous substitutes really work better and which one(s) work best.

**R. L. Ruberg, MD**

---

**Scar Lymphedema: Fact or Fiction?**
Warren AG, Slavin SA (Harvard Med School)
*Ann Plast Surg* 59:41-45, 2007

---

*Background.*—Few concepts are as fundamental to plastic surgery as scarring, yet swelling within a scar and its adjacent tissues is a common observation which is not well understood. Mechanical forces, scar contracture, fibrosis, and lymph stasis have been considered as possible explanations for these edematous-appearing areas, but conclusive evidence of a cause of swelling has not been established. The purpose of this study was to evaluate the possible role of microlymphatic stasis or disruption as a causal factor.

*Patients and Methods.*—Eleven patients (mean age: 43; range: 15 to 70) with localized swelling in conjunction with linear or curvilinear scars were evaluated, 9 with facial scars and 2 with scars of the chest wall and abdomen. Swelling within the scar had been present for an average of 4.5 years (range: 9 months to 13 years). Two patients had undergone previous Z-plasty revisions to the limbs of their curvilinear scars. Radiocolloid lymphoscintigraphy with technetium-99m $Sb_2S_3$ was performed on all patients by single or multiple injection technique into the site of the scar corresponding to local edema.

*Results.*—Following injection, rapid egress of radiotracer was visualized along lymphatic pathways posterior to the scar, with continuation to locoregional nodes in all patients with U-shaped "trapdoor" or linear scar configuration. However, in 8 cases there was no evidence of lymphatic drainage traversing or bridging the scar. In 2 patients with multiple prior Z-plasty revisions to the limbs of curvilinear scars, no visualization of lymph channels across the Z-plasty flaps was apparent. In total, 8 patients were diagnosed with lymphedema of the area adjacent to or enclosed within the scar.

*Conclusions.*—These findings suggest that undrained lymphatic fluid contributes to the pathogenesis of the raised and swollen tissues seen abutting a U-shaped scar. Furthermore, as lymphatic pathways do not reestablish themselves across scars, attempts at improving lymphatic flow with Z-plasty revisions may not succeed in patients with clinical trapdoor scar deformities. Determination of scar lymphedema can assist in the selection of proper management for patients seeking scar revision.

▶ I included this study because it demonstrates how experimental results and practical implementation may not match. The authors show clearly that in many patients with "trapdoor" or "biscuit" deformities, there are abnormalities of lymphatic reconnection. I guess that's not surprising, but the question is, "Does that mean that lymphatic drainage is critical for normal tissue contour?" I would say no, and in the discussion the authors agree. Since Z-plasty reconstruction fixes the overall majority of these deformities completely, it's hard to believe that the lack of lymphatic connections is important. So, the authors have proven that there are no lymphatic connections, but that doesn't matter. This article reminds us that simply documenting an abnormality or fact doesn't mean that it is the cause of a patient's problems or symptoms.

**W. L. Garner, MD**

---

### Pulsed Magnetic Fields Accelerate Cutaneous Wound Healing in Rats
Strauch B, Patel MK, Navarro JA, et al (Albert Einstein College of Medicine, New York; Columbia Univ, New York; Mount Sinai School of Medicine, New York)
*Plast Reconstr Surg* 120:425-430, 2007

---

*Background.*—Previous studies of pulsed magnetic fields have reported enhanced fracture and chronic wound healing, endothelial cell growth, and angiogenesis. This study characterizes the biomechanical changes that occur when standard cutaneous wounds are exposed to radiofrequency pulsed magnetic fields with specific dosage parameters, in an attempt to determine whether return to functional tensile strength could be accelerated in wound healing.

*Methods.*—There were two study phases and a total of 100 rats. In phase 1, wounds were exposed to a 1.0-G pulsed magnetic field signal in clinical use for wound repair for 30 minutes twice daily for 21 or 60 days. Phase 2 was a prospective, placebo-controlled, double-blind trial in which rats were treated for 30 minutes twice daily with three different low-amplitude signals (0.02 to 0.05 G), configured assuming a $Ca^{2+}$ binding transduction pathway, for 21 days. A midline, 8-cm, linear skin incision was made on the rat dorsum. Tensile strength was determined by measuring the point of rupture of the wound on a standard tensiometer loaded at 0.45 mm/second.

*Results.*—The mean tensile strength of treated groups in phase 1 was 48 percent ($p < 0.001$) greater than that of controls at 21 days; there was no significant difference at 60 days. In phase 2, the treated groups showed 18 percent (not significant), 44 percent, and 59 percent ($p < 0.001$) increases in tensile strength over controls at 21 days.

*Conclusion.*—The authors successfully demonstrated that exposing wounds to pulsed magnetic fields of very specific configurations accelerated early wound healing in this animal model, as evidenced by significantly increased wound tensile strength at 21 days after wounding.

▶ This is one of those interesting science articles that it's good to keep abreast of because we may eventually see this in our practice. Pulsed magnetic fields have been shown to be effective in a wide variety of clinical situations and are well referenced by the authors. In this case, an experimental study showed that pulsed magnetic fields improve the rate of healing. The authors have told me that they work in patients and that they do use this in their clinical practice. Does it add value enough to justify increased cost? How does this work in high risk and impaired wound healing situations? These are all the questions that we need to ask and answer before any of us can decide whether or not this technology has meaning. But in the meantime, pulsed magnetic fields? Who knew?

**W. L. Garner, MD**

---

**Does Rat Granulation Tissue Maturation Involve Gap Junction Communications?**
Au K, Ehrlich HP (Milton S. Hershey Med Ctr, Hershey, PA)
*Plast Reconstr Surg* 120:91-99, 2007

---

*Background.*—Wound healing, a coordinated process, proceeds by sequential changes in cell differentiation and terminates with the deposition of a new connective tissue matrix, a scar. Initially, there is the migratory fibroblast, followed by the proliferative fibroblast, then the synthetic fibroblast, which transforms into the myofibroblast, and finally the apoptotic fibroblast. Gap junction intercellular communications are proposed to coordinate the stringent control of fibroblast phenotypic changes. Does added oleamide, a natural fatty acid that blocks gap junction intercellular communications, alter the phenotypic progression of wound fibroblasts?

*Methods.*—Pairs of polyvinyl alcohol sponges attached to Alzet pumps, which constantly pumped either oleamide or vehicle solvent, were implanted subcutaneously into three rats. On day 8, implants were harvested and evaluated histologically and biochemically.

*Results.*—The capsule of oleamide-treated sponge contained closely packed fibroblasts with little connective tissue between them. The birefringence intensity of that connective tissue was reduced, indicating a reduced density of collagen fiber bundles. Myofibroblasts, identified immunohisto-logically by $\alpha$-smooth muscle actin–stained stress fibers, were reduced in oleamide-treated implants. Western blot analysis showing less $\alpha$-smooth muscle actin confirmed the reduced density of myofibroblasts.

*Conclusions.*—It appears that oleamide retards the progression of wound repair, where less connective tissue is deposited, the collagen is less organized, and the appearance of myofibroblasts is impaired. These findings support the hypothesis that gap junction intercellular communications between wound fibroblasts in granulation tissue play a role in the progression of repair and the maturation of granulation tissue into scar.

▶ I must admit that I know Dr. Ehrlich well and continue to view his scientific advances with admiration and respect. In this case, Dr. Ehrlich looks at how a particular cell organelle (gap junctions) causes tissues to remodel and mature. I won't go into great length about the experimental details of this article, which I find interesting from a scientific viewpoint, but rather would suggest to the readers that it validates a very important quality of life, that is, as we mature we improve our communication skills. I know that's happened with me personally and the validation of this principle in the tissues of healing wounds makes me believe that it is a universal principle that we all should remember.

**W. L. Garner, MD**

# 8 Grafts, Flaps, and Microsurgery

---

**The keystone design perforator island flap. Part II: clinical applications**
Pelissier P, Gardet H, Pinsolle V, et al (Hôpital Pellegrin-Tondu, Bordeaux, France; Université Bordeaux, France; Collège Français de Chirurgie Dermatologique, Paris; et al)
*J Plast Reconstr Aesthetic Surg* 60:888-891, 2007

---

*Background.*—This curvilinear- and trapezoidal-shaped flap essentially consists of two conjoined V–Y flaps end to side. The vascular supply is supported by the subcutaneous vascular network and is dependent on fascial and muscular perforators. A review of 15 clinical cases was performed to assess the reliability and versatility of the flap.

*Methods.*—Twelve keystone flaps were performed following excision of skin tumours or post-traumatic defects in various locations, from the head and neck region, the trunk and the limbs.

*Results.*—No flap necrosis, even partial, was observed regardless of the site and the type of keystone used. Patients were almost pain free in the postoperative course. The aesthetic results are quite satisfactory, as the flap is aligned locally without evidence of the ʹpincushioningʹ appearance sometimes seen around island reconstructions.

*Discussion.*—Elevation of the flap seems to evenly distribute the tensional forces without undermining. The flap is particularly useful in the repair of defects following skin cancer removal. Bulk is not a problem and good skin cover is achieved.

*Conclusion.*—The presence of perforators and subcutaneous network distributed throughout the body create an environment which makes this flap universally applicable and extremely reliable.

▶ This flap is receiving increased clinical use throughout the field of plastic surgery. The authors reported an anatomic study in a companion article,[1] which summarizes its concept and implementation. If you haven't read about this procedure, I would recommend it strongly. We all sometimes forget that geometric reorganizations of tissue with intact blood supply can be useful procedures. I would recommend considering it and trying it out. This flap will get you out of many difficult reconstruction problems with less work than other procedures.

**W. L. Garner, MD**

*Reference*

1. Pelissier P, Santoul M, Pinsolle V, Casoli V, Behan F. The keystone design perforator island flap. Part I: anatomic study. *J Plast Reconstr Aesth Surg.* 2007;60: 883-887.

### The Internal Mammary Artery Perforator Flap: An Anatomical Study and a Case Report
Vesely MJJ, Murray DJ, Novak CB, et al (Univ of Toronto; Univ Health Network, Toronto)
*Ann Plast Surg* 58:156-161, 2007

The anatomic basis for the internal artery mammary perforator (IMAP) flap is described in this cadaveric study, together with a clinical case report. The IMAP flap is based on a single or double perforator of the internal mammary artery that is included in the pedicle for added length. It provides a very useful source of local tissue with skin of good texture and color for head and neck reconstruction and, being muscle free, is thin. With preservation of the anterior cutaneous branch of the intercostal nerve, the flap has the potential to be sensate. A large area can be covered, particularly if bilateral flaps are raised. The donor site can be closed directly. In selected patients, it offers an excellent option for use in head and neck reconstruction and should be considered as an alternative to the deltopectoral and pectoralis major flaps.

▶ This is an interesting variation of the deltopectoral flap, based on several different perforators of the internal mammary artery. Other variations of chest wall flaps have been presented in the literature since 1931.

The authors state that the advantages of this flap are that it reduces the need for a visible and unsightly skin graft, at the donor site necessary, when the deltopectoral flap is used, and the flap is less bulky than the pectoralis major flap. However, primary closure of the flap is likely to produce severe distortion of the chest and breast in men and women, respectively. Its reach into the neck is adequate, but without delay, it is not capable of resurfacing defects above the mandible. Safe dissection of the perforator's supplying flap will require the surgeon to resect the costal cartilage and have microsurgical experience.

**S. H. Miller, MD, MPH**

## Free Flap Reexploration: Indications, Treatment, and Outcomes in 1193 Free Flaps

Bui DT, Cordeiro PG, Hu Q-Y, et al (Mem Sloan-Kettering Cancer Ctr, New York)
*Plast Reconstr Surg* 119:2092-2100, 2007

*Background.*—Microvascular free tissue transfer is a reliable method for reconstruction of complex surgical defects. However, there is still a small risk of flap compromise necessitating urgent reexploration. A comprehensive study examining the causes and methods of avoiding or treating these complications has not been performed. The purpose of this study was to review the authors' experience with a large number of microvascular complications over an 11-year period.

*Methods.*—This was a retrospective review of all free flaps performed from 1991 to 2002 at Memorial Sloan-Kettering Cancer Center. All patients who required emergent reexploration were identified, and the incidence of vascular complications and methods used for their management were analyzed.

*Results.*—A total of 1193 free flaps were performed during the study period, of which 6 percent required emergent reexploration. The most common causes for reexploration were pedicle thrombosis (53 percent) and hematoma/bleeding (30 percent). The overall flap survival rate was 98.8 percent. Venous thrombosis was more common than arterial thrombosis (74 versus 26 percent) and had a higher salvage rate (71 versus 40 percent). Salvaged free flaps were reexplored more quickly than failed flaps (4 versus 9 hours after detection; $p = 0.01$). There was no significant difference in salvage rate in flaps requiring secondary vein grafting or thrombolysis as compared with those with anastomotic revision only.

*Conclusions.*—Microvascular free tissue transfer is a reliable reconstructive technique with low failure rates. Careful monitoring and urgent reexploration are critical for salvage of compromised flaps. The majority of venous thromboses can be salvaged. Arterial thromboses can be more problematic. An algorithm for flap exploration and salvage is presented.

▶ The Sloan-Kettering group has looked at their free flap experience and analyzed their indications, treatment, and outcomes of free flap re-exploration. I recommend the article as a superb and well-documented review. More importantly though, I recommend their algorithm. Anytime a group with this experience critically assesses their results, we must take note. The process is clear and simple, supported by their data. We will certainly endorse this process in our program. As important, I compliment them for not simply analyzing their data, but transferring that experience to outcomes. We need more of this type of review.

**D. J. Smith, Jr, MD**

# 9 Other Topics in Plastic and Aesthetic Surgery

**Influence of Povidone-Iodine Preoperative Showers on Skin Colonization in Elective Plastic Surgery Procedures**
Veiga DF, Damasceno CAV, Filho JV, et al (Universidade do Vale do Sapucaí, Pouso Alegre, Brazil; Universidade Federal de São Paulo)
*Plast Reconstr Surg* 121:115-118, 2008

*Background.*—Preoperative showering with antiseptic skin cleansers is common in elective operations, although the value of this procedure in reducing surgical wound infections has not been established. The authors designed a prospective study to assess the influence of povidone-iodine preoperative showers on skin colonization in elective plastic surgery procedures.

*Methods.*—Patients, older than 18 years, scheduled for elective and clean plastic surgery procedures on the thorax or abdomen were assigned, randomly, to the povidone-iodine group ($n = 57$) or to a control group ($n = 57$). Patients allocated to the povidone-iodine group took a shower with liquid detergent–based povidone-iodine 10%, 2 hours before surgery. For the control group, no special instructions for showering were implemented before surgery. Quantitative skin cultures were obtained just before the preoperative scrub in the operating room. Samples were plated on hypertonic mannitol agar, blood agar, Sabouraud agar with chloramphenicol, and eosin-methylene blue agar. Samples were collected and processed, and results were assessed by blinded investigators

*Results.*—Staphylococcal skin colonization was significantly lower in the povidone-iodine group ($p < 0.001$). No microorganism growth was observed on 33 percent of the postshower skin cultures from patients in the povidone-iodine shower group, compared with 0 percent of the cultures from patients in the control group. Colonies of fungi and enterobacteria were recovered in small amounts in both groups, and povidone-iodine showers did not significantly reduce skin colonization by these microorganisms.

*Conclusion.*—Single preoperative povidone-iodine showers are effective in reducing staphylococcal skin colonization before elective, clean plastic surgical procedures on the thorax and abdomen.

▶ In the 1950s, when *Staphylococcus aureus* infections were just beginning to blossom, the standard surgical preparation was a shave the night before with reusable razors, which were somewhat dull and painted with a tincture of iodine, which caused irritation in itself. In addition, they wrapped the area or the limb with a sterile towel, which produced a wonderful environment for bacterial proliferation. In the morning, folliculitis became commonplace, as did cancellations of elective cases. We learned to omit shaving of patients from the neurosurgical service. Interestingly, at that time, they had adapted the practice not because of folliculitis, but because of the possibility of the demise of the patient overnight, due to the severity of the neurosurgical medical condition. If the head had been shaved, this could create some problems in an expired patient. We adopted their practice and shaved just before the procedure, or not at all, and found less infections. The addition of a nontraumatic scrub 2 hours before surgery makes a good deal of sense, since infection is a matter of host resistance, tissue trauma, and the number of bacteria.

**P. W. McKinney, MD, CM**

---

### Resumption of Sexual Activity after Plastic Surgery: Current Practice and Recommendations

Rankin M, Borah G, Alvarez S (Rutgers Univ, New Brunswick, NJ; Univ of Medicine and Dentistry of New Jersey, New Brunswick)
*Plast Reconstr Surg* 120:1557-1563, 2007

---

*Background.*—Information on sexual counseling and practice guidelines after plastic surgery is quite limited and poorly documented as part of clinical care after surgery. The aim of this study was to assess board-certified plastic surgeons' current practices and to make clinical recommendations for resumption of sexual activity in the postoperative period.

*Methods.*—A descriptive mailed survey of randomly chosen American Society of Plastic Surgeons' members was designed to evaluate plastic surgeons' methods of screening for sexual concerns, the frequency of postoperative discussions with patients, and clinical recommendations for safe sexual positions.

*Results.*—There were 281 respondents, for a response rate of 40 percent. A minority of plastic surgeons (32.9 percent) felt it was the surgeon's role to provide postoperative sexual counseling regarding restrictions and guidelines; the majority of plastic surgeons (63 percent) felt that their nurse should provide this service. Patients never (46.6 percent) or rarely (23.8 percent) asked about sexual activity restrictions after surgery. Some surgeons (27.8 percent) proactively discussed postoperative sexual activity, but 57.3 percent said they rarely or never gave specific advice. There were gender differences; male plastic surgeons discussed specific sexual techniques and positions significantly more frequently than female plastic surgeons ($p = 0.001$), and patients ask male plastic surgeons significantly more frequently about sexual activity restrictions than they do female plastic surgeons ($p = 0.001$).

*Conclusions.*—Many plastic surgeons gave little or no advice to patients regarding resumption of sexual activity after surgery, and the majority of patients do not initiate the discussion. Most surgeons expect their nursing staff to provide sexual counseling.

▶ Sexual activity raises the blood pressure because of the physical exertion required. A hematoma 1 week after surgery usually represents stress/exertion from a number of possible sources. Rarely will a patient offer sex as the reason, but there is a beautiful antidote years ago by Dr Owlsley, who related that he had a patient whose husband admired the result so much that he could not wait any more, and she required the removal of the resultant hematoma 1 week after the operation.

**P. W. McKinney, MD, CM**

---

### Body Dysmorphic Disorder: Diagnosis and Approach
Jakubietz M, Jakubietz RJ, Kloss DF, et al (Kantonsspital St Gallen, Switzerland)
*Plast Reconstr Surg* 119:1924-1930, 2007

---

Body dysmorphic disorder is a psychiatric disease that can be frequently encountered in an aesthetic practice. Body dysmorphic disorder is characterized by a preoccupation with a minimal or nonexistent appearance defect, and it causes significant distress and interferes with the social life of the patient. The perceived physical anomaly may involve the shape and size of the whole body or may be centered around single units. Body dysmorphic disorder patients are known to request multiple aesthetic procedures that leave them unsatisfied. Only a timely diagnosis will enable the surgeon and staff to adequately address the patient's needs. Body dysmorphic disorder patients cannot be cured with surgery. Diagnostic techniques, such as patient interview and observation, are presented in this article. With this, the plastic surgeon should be able to diagnose body dysmorphic disorder, preoperatively. Using the presented algorithm to approach body dysmorphic disorder patients, will avoid disappointment for patients and surgeons alike.

▶ Maximum distress for a minimal deformity should ring the alarms—Mark Gorney emphasized this principle over 20 years ago, and it is germane to this distressing abnormality, which disrupts the patient's life and the doctor's practice. It is mostly a "hunch," which becomes clearer afterwards; with experience, one can minimize the chances of operating these patients. Multiple surgeries and maximal distress for a minimal deformity, all in a seemingly rational patient, should raise the possibility of body dysmorphic disorder.

**P. W. Mckinney, MD, CM**

---

**Von Willebrand Disease: Screening, Diagnosis, and Management**
Totonchi A, Eshraghi Y, Beck D, et al (Case Western Reserve Univ, Cleveland, OH)
*Aesthet Surg J* 28:189-194, 2008

---

Von Willebrand disease (vWD), a hemorrhagic disorder mimicking a defect in platelet function, is the most commonly inherited coagulopathy, resulting in a deficiency that may prolong bleeding time and increase risk for major bleeding complications during surgery. Von Willebrand factor (vWF) serves a dual role in hemostasis: mediating the initial platelet adhesion to damaged endothelium at the site of vessel injury and stabilizing coagulation factor VIII, an important cofactor in the generation of a fibrin clot. Although quantitative or qualitative defects in vWF protein can manifest as a mild to severe bleeding disorder, many cases of vWD remain subclinical, barring major invasive stimuli, and undetected by either patient or clinician. Nevertheless, the frequency of this coagulation disorder would almost ensure that every plastic surgeon will encounter affected patients, making a thorough understanding of vWD and its management absolutely necessary. Surprisingly, there is little information concerning vWD in the plastic surgery literature. Our goal is to familiarize the plastic surgeon with vWD, including physiology, diagnostic criteria, classification, and molecular basis for multiple vWD variants, and diagnosis and management.

▶ My first encounter with Von Willebrand's disease was in the recovery room after my first solo cleft palate repair as a resident at The New York Hospital. My elegant push-back repair would not cease bleeding. In 1965, even less was known of the coagulopathy than now. At the recommendation of our junior attending, Dr Goulian, we took turns holding pressure directly on the repair in the recovery room in this nearly 2-year-old patient. "Gently," I cautioned the intern. It did stop bleeding that evening, and the repair did not dehisce. We had vague recollection of the literature, such as family history and patient's personal history, but little was known of this entity except for the family history and to apply direct pressure. We consulted with the relatively new specialty of hematology; but by then, the bleeding had stopped. I subsequently encountered this defect 3 additional times in my career, or about every 15 years. Each time, the treatment got more sophisticated and proactive. The author's review brings us up to date on how to avoid a day in the recovery room.

**P. W. McKinney, MD, CM**

## Thromboembolic prophylaxis in plastic surgery: a 12-year follow up in the UK

Conroy FJ, Thornton DJA, Mather DP, et al (Castle Hill Hosp, Cottingham, Hull, England)
*J Plast Reconstr Aesthetic Surg* 59:510-514, 2006

Potentially fatal thromboembolic events prevail post-operatively, despite the widespread availability of proven methods of prophylaxis. In 1992, Dujon et al published an article which reviewed thromboembolic prophylaxis methods of Consultant Plastic Surgeons in the UK and Ireland.

Our follow up study surveyed all current Consultant B.A.P.S members using a modified postal questionnaire to assess practice nationwide. Our conclusions were drawn from comparisons made between the two populations some twelve years apart.

Our results show a dramatic change from the previous findings. Since 1992 86% of respondents have developed a set prophylaxis protocol (compared to 19%). The use of low molecular weight heparin has drastically increased by 24% to 76%, the use of flow-tron boots (or similar) has increased by 22% to 68%, the use of TED stockings has increased by 12% to 83%, the use of multi-modality prophylaxis has increased by 27% to 79%.

Our results demonstrate a definite shift towards multi-modal thromboembolic prophylaxis, possibly due to increased awareness of available technologies and subsequent reduction in costs (Table 1).

▶ Table 1 reminds us of ASPS guidelines. The authors emphasize the current modalities of prevention. In rhitidectomy, for example, preoperative preparation

TABLE 1.—American Society of Plastic Surgery Task Force On Deep Vein Thrombosis Prophylaxis Guidelines

|  | Risk Factors | Recommendations |
|---|---|---|
| Low risk | No known risk factors | Comfortable positioning |
|  | Under 40 years of age | Slight knee flexion (to aid popliteal venous return) |
|  | Procedure lasting <30 min |  |
| Moderate risk | Over 40 years of age | As above PLUS |
|  | Procedure lasting >30 min | Intermittent pneumatic compression garments worn in the pre-, peri-, and post-op periods until patient fully mobile |
|  | Patient on OCP or HRT | All 'risky' medications to be stopped |
| High risk | Over 40 years of age | As above PLUS |
|  | Procedure lasting >30 min | Pre-op haematology consultation |
|  | Patient on OCP or HRT | Consideration for LMWH 2 h prior to surgery and daily until patient is fully mobile |
|  | Obesity | (Prophylactic anticoagulation is optional in procedures with a high risk of haematoma) |
|  | Malignancy |  |
|  | Immobilisation |  |
|  | Hypercoaguable states |  |

that is, weight control, exercise, diet, and avoidance coupled with the intraoperative use of compression boots should be used. In addition, expeditious surgery minimizes the operative risks.

**P. W. McKinney, MD, CM**

---

**Factors Impacting Thromboembolism after Bariatric Body Contouring Surgery**
Shermak MA, Chang DC, Heller J (Johns Hopkins Med Institutions, Baltimore, MD)
*Plast Reconstr Surg* 119:1590-1598, 2007

---

*Background.*—The purpose of this study was to define the risk of venous thromboembolism within the massive weight loss population undergoing body contouring procedures.

*Methods.*—Retrospective analysis of massive weight loss patients who had body contouring operations, between March of 1998 and September of 2004, was performed. Patient factors studied included age, gender, medical comorbidities including history of thromboembolic complications, depression, tobacco use, preoperative/postoperative body mass index, surgery, and transfusion.

*Results.*—There were 138 cases, and the female-to-male ratio was 5:1. Procedures were often combined: 128 patients had abdominal surgery, 36 had a back lift, 41 had brachioplasty, 29 had chest surgery, and 47 had a thigh lift. The most common complications were related to healing ($n = 28$) and seroma ($n = 18$). Three patients had postoperative deep venous thrombosis requiring anticoagulation, and one had a fatal pulmonary embolism, making the overall venous thromboembolism risk 2.9 percent. The mean body mass index at contour was 48.5 for patients with venous thromboembolism versus 31.8 for patients who did not develop venous thromboembolism ($p = 0.01$). Looking at this subgroup of 45 patients, the risk of venous thromboembolism was 8.9 percent, with no risk found in patients with a body mass index less than 35 ($p = 0.01$).

*Conclusions.*—The risk of venous thromboembolism with contouring surgery for massive weight loss is comparable to that for gastric bypass surgery. Body mass index in the obese range appears to be a leading risk factor. The authors' data support routine prophylaxis against venous thromboembolism. Recommendations for high-risk patients are discussed.

▶ The higher the body mass index (especially over 35), the greater the risk for venous thromboembolism in body contouring. Prophylaxis (anticoagulants, compression boots, preoperative conditioning, and early ambulation) is helpful. Shortened operating times, rather than an overly ambitious undertaking, is also paramount to reduce this risk.

**P. W. McKinney, MD, CM**

## The Surgeon's Role and Responsibility in Facial Tissue Allograft Transplantation

Sacks JM, Keith JD, Fisher C, et al (Univ of Pittsburgh, PA)
*Ann Plast Surg* 58:595-601, 2007

Facial composite tissue allograft (CTA) transplantation represents a novel frontier in the reconstruction of the human form. The face plays a central role in human interactions, with significant social ramifications resulting from facial disfigurement. The surgeon performing facial tissue transplantation bears additional responsibilities unique to plastic and reconstructive procedures. Reconstruction by facial tissue transplantation may immensely improve quality of life, provided the process of patient selection is conspicuous and appropriate, and allograft rejection is prevented. However, facial CTA transplantation represents an elective procedure to reconstruct a non–life-threatening defect. Given the potential for organ failure, opportunistic infection and malignancy, resulting from long-term immunosuppression, the surgeon must carefully weigh the balance of risk to benefit for the individual patient. Pioneering surgeons, developing this procedure, must thoroughly evaluate its impact, as it relates to clinical and social issues.

▶ The authors present a thoughtful and balanced, albeit cautious, discussion regarding a plastic surgeon's role in facial transplantation. It offers the reader the opportunity to review the possible indications, potential benefits, and risks of the procedure as they relate to immunosuppressive therapy and failure of the graft. The references are quite extensive and should be helpful to any plastic surgeon interested in learning more about this procedure. Especially worthwhile is the paper by Freedman.[1]

The authors suggest, in their opinion, that it is the responsibility of the medical profession to balance ethics with innovation, as it educates and shapes society's perceptions of, and interests in, new procedures. It is the accountability of this type that epitomizes the essence of professionalism. Their call for a multidisciplinary approach echoes the wisdom espoused by Nobel Laureate Joseph E. Murray.

**S. H. Miller, MD, MPH**

*Reference*

1. Freedman B. Equipoise and the ethics of clinical research. *N Engl J Med.* 1987; 317:141-145.

**Plastic Surgery Classics: Characteristics of 50 Top-Cited Articles in Four Plastic Surgery Journals since 1946**
Loonen MPJ, Hage JJ, Kon M (Univ Med Ctr Utrecht, The Netherlands)
*Plast Reconstr Surg* 121:320e-327e, 2008

*Background.*—Citation of published articles by peers provides an indication of the relevance of the scientific work. Still, it is unknown what kinds of plastic surgery articles are cited most often. The authors set out to identify the characteristics of the 50 top-cited articles as published in four international, peer-reviewed, PubMed-indexed general plastic surgery journals.

*Methods.*—The 50 most-cited articles were identified in each of the following journals: *Plastic and Reconstructive Surgery*, the *British Journal of Plastic Surgery*, the *Annals of Plastic Surgery*, and the *Scandinavian Journal of Plastic and Reconstructive Surgery and Hand Surgery*. These 200 articles were ranked after their citation index, defined as the mean number of times they were cited per year during the first 16 years after publication. The top-50 articles thus ranked were analyzed for citation and journal distribution, geographic and institutional origin, surgical and anatomical subject, and level of evidence.

*Results.*—Forty-one of the 50 top-cited articles (82 percent) were published in *Plastic and Reconstructive Surgery* and 35 articles (70 percent) originated from institutions within the United States. Most of the articles dealt with the reconstruction of acquired defects (45 percent) and with basic or experimental research (41 percent). Research that offered means for clinical improvement, rather than a high level of evidence or the results of multi-institutional collaboration, was most often cited.

*Conclusion.*—An article featuring a clinical or nonclinical innovation, observation, or discovery that leads to clinical improvement has the best potential to become a "classic."

▶ This is a fascinating look at the world of plastic surgical literature, at least as recorded in English and spanning the years 1946-2000. The use of a citation index, mean number of citations per year up to 16 years since publication, seems far more reliable than the total number of citations. However, one must recognize that the Science Citation Index Expanded database (ISI Thompson Scientific) covers more than 6000 journals, but primarily those published in English. Would the results have been similar had the authors also counted citations in books? Another area of relative importance for future studies such as these will, no doubt, include electronic citations. Were one to look at these results longitudinally, would the heavy American presence on these lists continue? I applaud the authors' call for more multi-institutional collaborative studies, as I believe that can reduce some of the problems associated with relatively low levels of evidence.

**S. H. Miller, MD, MPH**

**Implementation and Evaluation of a New Surgical Residency Model**
Schneider JR, Coyle JJ, Ryan ER, et al (Northwestern Univ, Chicago)
*J Am Coll Surg* 205:393-404, 2007

*Background.*—The Accreditation Council for Graduate Medical Education (ACGME) duty-hour requirements prompted program directors to rethink the organizational structure of their residency programs. Many surgical educators have expressed concerns that duty-hour restrictions would negatively affect quality of resident education. This article summarizes evaluation research results collected to study the impact of our reengineered residency program designed to preserve important educational activities while meeting duty-hour accreditation requirements.

*Study Design.*—The traditional residency structure was redesigned to include a mixture of apprenticeship, small team, and night-float models. Impact evaluation data were collected using operative case logs, standardized test scores, quality assurance data, resident perception surveys, a faculty survey, and process evaluation measures.

*Results.*—PGY1s and PGY2s enjoyed a substantial increase in operative cases. Operative cases increased overall and no resident has failed to meet ACGME volume or distribution requirements. American Board of Surgery In-Training Examination performance improved for PGY1s and PGY2s. Patient outcomes measures, including monthly mortality and number of and charges for admissions, showed no changes. Anonymously completed rotation evaluation forms showed stable or improved resident perceptions of case load, continuity, operating room teaching, appropriate level of faculty involvement and supervision, encouragement to attend conferences, and general assessment of the learning environment. A quality-of-life survey completed by residents before and after implementation of the new program structure showed substantial improvements. Faculty surveys showed perceived increases in work hours and job dissatisfaction. New physician assistant and nurse positions directly attributed to duty-hour restrictions amounted to about 0.2 full-time equivalent per resident.

*Conclusions.*—Duty-hour restrictions produce new challenges and might require additional resources but need not cause a deterioration of surgical residents' educational experience.

▶ It is unusual to include an abstract on surgical education with these reviews. There is no clinical lesson to be learned, but there are enormous surgical implications. Most think that just residency program directors and academicians will be interested. On the contrary, everyone should take note because this reflects the changing landscapes of surgery. Competencies that are being used in the residencies are and will be competencies in the maintenance of certification. The residencies are more compact and easier to evaluate. For those of you looking for associates and partners, it will be important to understand the paradigm shift in training. There is clearly a difference in training today. It is important to understand the evolution.

**D. J. Smith, Jr, MD**

## Wound Education: American Medical Students Are Inadequately Trained in Wound Care

Patel NP, Granick MS (Univ of Medicine and Dentistry of New Jersey–New Jersey Med School, Newark, NJ)
Ann Plast Surg 59:53-55, 2007

Millions of patients are treated annually in the United States with either acute or chronic wounds, costing billions of dollars. This is a retrospective study designed to quantify the directed education that medical students receive in their 4 years of training on 3 wound-related topics: physiology of tissue injury, physiology of wound healing, and clinical wound healing. The mean hours of education in physiology of tissue injury at 50 American medical schools are 0.5 hours and 0.2 hours, respectively, in the first year and second years and none in the third and fourth years. The mean hours of directed education in the physiology of wound healing are 2.1 hours and 1.9 hours in the first and second years. The data in our study show there is scant directed education in relevant wound topics in American medical schools. Considering the immense economic and social impact of wounds in our society, more attention should be paid to the education of our physician trainees on this important topic.

▶ Dr. Granick and colleagues review the curriculum of United States Medical Schools, which that among the hundreds of hours of education they receive through the 4 years of schooling, only an average of 9 hours are spent on wound healing. This is a ridiculously small amount, in view of the likelihood that every practitioner will be caring for patients with wounds. It shows a profound imbalance with the likelihood of treating someone with syndromic endocrine problems or inborn errors of metabolism presenting in childhood. This lack of relevance is significant and it is probably our job as wound healing experts to step up and begin demanding that our schools provide this education.

I'm not sure this is the right audience to present this article, because plastic surgeons are, in general, wound healing providers. If we educated our family practice, internal medicine, and other surgical colleagues, we would likely get fewer consults. However, that would probably be best for patients.

**W. L. Garner, MD**

## Assessment of the microsurgical skills: 30 minutes versus 2 weeks patency

Ilie V, Ilie V, Ghetu N, et al ("Gr.T. Popa" Univ of Medicine, Iasi, Romania)
Microsurgery 27:451-454, 2007

The aim of this study is to evaluate the amount of training needed by a trainee, with no background in microsurgery, in order to achieve proper skills for microvascular anastomosis. A protocol based on the rat femoral artery was established to provide a quantitative representation. Five inexperienced subjects started performing microvascular anastomosis. Patency was assessed at 30 min. The final assessment was performed at 2 weeks when rats were reoperated and the patency below the anastomosis was checked. The experiment was discontinued for one subject when he/she succeeded to have two series of four anastomosis with 100% patency at 2 weeks. The results were: 47.5% patency rate at 30 min and 7.5% at 2 weeks (series 1–2); 67.5 and 32.5% (3–4); 82.5 and 35% (5–6); 100 and 70% (7–8); 100 and 87.5% (9–10). Two trainees obtained 100% patency at 2 weeks after series 9–10. Other three needed two more series. There is a significant statistic difference ($P < 0.01$) between the results at 30 min and 2 weeks for the series (1–2, 3–4, 5–6, 7–8). The patency rate at 2 weeks reflects in a better way the microsurgical skills of a trainee. For long term functioning anastomosis, the training period needs an extension beyond that necessary for 100% patency at 30 min.

▶ I'm always glad to see articles that look at how to train our residents, because we seldom study this enough. In this case, the authors are investigating how to train inexperienced surgeons to do microsurgery. They document effectively that 2-week patency is a better outcome measure than 30 minutes. This is not surprising, I guess, and is more clinically relevant and would be a good idea. However, this then requires the microsurgical course director to obtain animal care approval, requires survival surgery, and will immensely increase the costs of this training. Whether this is good or bad is not clear to me. Although, I would estimate that it would cost in excess of $100 to keep these rats alive for the 2 weeks needed to assess 2-week patency. Whether or not this is worth it, I am not sure.

**W. L. Garner, MD**

# Subject Index

latissimus dorsi
  for reconstruction of complex chest
    wall defects, 23
  reinnervated myocutaneous, for total
    phalloplasty in female-to-male
    transsexuals, 30
  lower abdominal free, for unilateral
    breast reconstruction, 190
  medial sural artery perforator, for tongue
    and floor of mouth reconstruction,
    13
  pectoralis major muscle, for complete
    obliteration of median sternotomy
    wound, 21
  perforator-sparing buttock rotation for
    coverage of pressure sores, 25
  for reconstruction after sternal wound
    infection, 20
  rectus abdominis transposition with
    intercostal artery pedicle for sternal
    wound reconstruction, 22
Fractures
  facial, financial analysis of operative
    management, 33
  medial orbital with entrapment, 34
Free flaps
  bilateral lower abdominal, for breast
    reconstruction, 190
  jejunal, for reconstruction after
    pharyngolaryngoesophagectomy, 14
  for lower limb salvage, failure rates, 39
  reexploration for salvage of, 207
  salvage treatments following failure
    caused by vascular thrombosis, in
    head and neck reconstruction, 18

## G

Gluteal augmentation
  indications and surgical management,
    130
Gracilis muscle flap
  for coverage of groin wounds, 27
  unilateral myofasciocutaneous
    advancement, for single-stage
    reconstruction of scrotal and
    perineal defects, 27
Groin wounds
  gracilis muscle flap for coverage of, 27

## H

Hairline
  anterior temporal, follicular anatomy
    and its implications for
    rhytidectomy, 100

Hand
  arterialized venous flaps for
    reconstruction, 62
  contracture after burn injury, flap choices
    for, 49
  current practice of microsurgery by
    members of the American Society
    for Surgery of the Hand, 61
  functional gracilis flap in thenar
    reconstruction, 60
Head and neck reconstruction
  free jejunal flaps for reconstruction after
    pharyngolaryngoesophagectomy,
    14
  free-tissue transfer for
    economic factors affecting use of, 15
    influence of medical complications on
      morbidity, mortality, and true costs,
      19
  medial sural artery perforator flap for
    tongue and mouth of floor
    reconstruction, 13
  microvascular free flaps, cartilage
    grafts, and a paramedian forehead
    flap for aesthetic reconstruction
    of the nose and adjacent facial
    units, 16
  outcomes of primary versus secondary
    mandibular reconstruction in, 10
  reconstruction of orbital floor and
    maxilla with divided vascularized
    calvarial bone flap in one session,
    11
  salvage treatments following failure of
    free flap transfer caused by vascular
    thrombosis, 18
Head and neck trauma
  financial analysis of operative facial
    fracture management, 33
  nasolacrimal duct reconstruction with
    nasal mucoperiosteal flap, 35
  white-eyed medial blowout fracture, 34
Human immunodeficiency virus (HIV)
  lipodystrophy associated with, plastic
    surgical options for, 133
Hypertrophic scars
  postoperative radiation protocol for,
    193
  topical silicone gel elastomers for, 195

## I

Implants, breast
  cancer risk in women with, 177
  filling beyond manufacturer's
    recommended fill volume, 174

# Author Index